# THE MENOPAUSE WEIGHT LOSS DIET

The Ultimate Menopause Guide with Over 100 Delicious and Simple Recipes for Natural and Efficient Weight Loss for Women Over 50. 21-day Meal Plan and Journal.

Belinda Smith

# Table of Contents

# INTRODUCTION

As women age, health becomes a primary topic to be discussed all the time as women undergo a lot of bodily changes, an important one being the changes that come with the menopause stage.

**Menopause** is the period when a woman stops getting monthly menstrual flow tagged 'period'. It happens when the ovaries stop producing and releasing eggs every month. When this happens, women are no longer able to get pregnant and give birth biologically. It also marks the time when a woman's menstrual cycles come to an end. Usually, It is diagnosed after a woman fails to menstruate for 12 months.

However, menopause is not a disease nor a disorder, for you to be scared of, it is rather, a completely natural biological process that occurs amongst all women and It is part of the transition stage of women into old age. At this stage, women are usually preoccupied with other things going on in their lives. They may be caring for aging parents or relatives, supporting their children as they also transition into adulthood and teenagers, or undertaking major responsibilities in their job and place of employment. So, it's not a disability.

The age range for menopause in women varies from one region to the other. According to studies, most women experience menopause in their 40s or 50s; however, it occurs at an average age of 51 in the United States.
This condition can last for a few months to several years or forever. However, many factors, including genetics and ovarian health, influence the age when women may enter menopause.
Menopause is preceded by perimenopause. **Perimenopause** is the period during which your hormones begin to change in preparation for menopause. It may occur for several months to years. Perimenopause usually strikes many women above 49 years of age while other women skip perimenopause entirely and hit menopause abruptly. During perimenopause, menstrual cycles become inconsistent. Your periods could be late, or you could entirely skip one or more of them, and the flow might also change from heavy to light.

**Premature menopause**, also known as primary ovarian insufficiency, affects about 1% of women before the age of 40 while menopause affects about 5% of women between the ages of 40 and 45. This term is known as early menopause. Every woman's menopausal experience is different. When menopause arrives quickly or over a short period, symptoms are frequently more severe. Conditions that affect ovarian health, such as cancer or hysterectomy, as well as certain lifestyle choices, such as smoking, are likely to enhance the severity and length of symptoms.

Symptoms of menopause vary from woman to woman. While some women are unaffected by menopausal symptoms and may even feel happy that they no longer have to worry about getting unpleasant periods or becoming pregnant, others get really affected by it. The degree to which they are affected depends on their body system. While some women may experience only one symptom, others experience a combination of the symptoms.

**Some of these symptoms include**:

- Reduced fertility

  Estrogen levels begin to diminish as a female near the end of her reproductive period but before menopause. This diminishes the likelihood of becoming pregnant.

- Menstruation irregularity

  Periods becoming less regular is usually the first symptom that menopause is approaching. They could arrive more frequently or less frequently than normal, and they could be heavier or lighter.

- Dryness and pain in the cervix

  Perimenopause can cause vaginal dryness, itching, and discomfort, which can last into menopause. Chafing and discomfort may occur during vaginal sex if any of these symptoms are present. Furthermore, if the skin cracks, the danger of infection increases.

- Vaginal atrophy, a disease characterized by vaginal wall weakening, dryness, and inflammation, can occur following menopause. Vaginal dryness and related disorders can be relieved with various moisturizers, lubricants, and drugs.

- Hot flashes

  Hot flashes are prevalent during the menopause period. They induce an unexpected sensation of heat in the upper torso. The sensation could begin in the face, neck, or chest and move upward or downward.
  The frequency of heat flashes varies greatly amongst people. For example, they can occur many times every hour, a few times per day, or less than once per week. Some people might even notice that their hot flashes follow a pattern.

  Blood arteries in the upper body enlarge during a hot flash, allowing increased blood flow to the area. This increased blood flow can result in blotchy skin patches or flushing. During the process, some people might feel anxious and stressed, especially if they are out in public and are worried about appearing flushed.
  As the body strives to cool itself after a hot flash, some may experience sweating that causes them to feel cold or shudder. Sweating also causes red spots to appear on the skin.

  In addition to or lieu of hot flashes, some persons have nocturnal sweats and cold flashes, or chills.

  Hot flashes typically appear within the first year after menopause, but they can also last for up to 14 years.

- Sleeplessness

  Sleep issues can emerge during menopause and can be caused by anxiety, night sweats, and an increased desire to urinate.

- Emotional changes

  Depression, anxiety, and low mood are all frequent symptoms of menopause. It is not uncommon to have periods of anger and weeping bouts.

  These problems can be worsened by hormonal fluctuations and sleep disruptions. A person's feelings regarding menopause may also play a role. Distress over poor libido or the cessation of fertility, for example, might lead to depression throughout menopause.

While sadness, anger, and fatigue are typical throughout menopause, they may not always imply depression. Nevertheless, once you start feeling in a low mood for more than two weeks, professional attention is required.

- Difficulties in learning and focusing.

During the buildup of menopause, many women do struggle with attention and memory.

Nevertheless, keeping yourself physically and mentally active, eating a healthy diet, and participating in social activities can all help with these concerns. You can decide to pick up a new activity, or hobby or join a club or a local activity to keep yourself active.

- Changes within the body.

Around the time of menopause, a variety of bodily changes might occur. Some people may encounter: fat accumulation in the abdomen weight gain changes in hair color and texture, decrease in breast volume as well as breast tenderness, and incontinence of the bladder - a problem associated with the muscles and nerves that help the bladder hold or pass urine, resulting in sudden and strong urge to urinate. It might also lead to leaky urines.

These bodily changes may occur independent of menopause and can be a result of it. They are not clear indications of menopause.

- Increased risk of certain medical conditions

The risk of various health concerns appears to rise after menopause. Though these illnesses are not caused by menopause, hormonal changes in the body might result in them. some of these diseases include:

- Osteoporosis: It is a long-term disorder characterized by a decline in bone strength and density. To preserve bone strength, a doctor may advise taking vitamin D pills and consuming more calcium-rich foods.

- Cardiovascular disease: Studies by the American Heart Association (AHA) has shown that a decrease in estrogen level in a woman due to menopause may raise the risk of cardiovascular disease. Even hormone therapy is not enough to lessen this risk.

- Breast cancer: Some kinds of breast cancer occur more frequently after menopause. Though menopause does not cause breast cancer, the hormonal changes that occur appear to increase the risk.

# NATURAL CAUSES OF MENOPAUSE

As earlier stated, menopause is a normal and natural process in an adult woman, in which the ovaries generate fewer reproductive hormones as they age. When the body doesn't supply enough hormones, then the body begins to undergo these changes to adjust the body. The hormones responsible for menopause includes:

- Estrogen
- Progesterone
- Testosterone
- luteinizing hormone (LH)
- Follicle-stimulating hormone (FSH)

The loss of active ovarian follicles is one of the most significant changes in women's bodies. Ovarian follicles are the structures in the ovarian wall that generate and release eggs, permitting menstruation and fertility.

Most women initially feel their period becomes less regular as the flow becomes heavier and longer. This normally happens between the ages of 40 and 50. However, most women in the United States have reached menopause by the age of 52.

# THE FOUR STAGES OF MENOPAUSE

Throughout a woman's life, her reproductive health varies dramatically. Hormones change dramatically during the reproductive years, from the first menstrual cycle through menopause and beyond, making each stage different.

Overall, the women's health cycle can be divided into four major stages.

## PRE-MENOPAUSE PERIOD

A woman in pre-menopause has a regular menstrual cycle, is in her peak reproductive years, and has no apparent symptoms of menopause. A woman is technically in the pre-menopause stage at any point before entering perimenopause.

## PERIMENOPAUSE STAGE

Perimenopause is a stage that occurs between pre-menopause and menopause. This stage usually begins in a woman's forties and lasts several years.

During this time, the effects of hormonal shifts will be visible as the ovaries gradually quit working. Common perimenopause symptoms such as the following frequently occur since estrogen synthesis slows and fewer eggs are released:

- Periods are becoming shorter and more irregular,
- Regular mood swings,
- Reduced sexual urge,
- Night sweats and hot flashes,
- Dryness of the cervix,
- Headaches,
- Concentration problems or brain fog,
- Muscle or joint pain, e.t.c.

While fertility is lowered and reproduction is less likely during perimenopause, a woman can still become pregnant.

## MENOPAUSE STAGE

Menopause can affect women between the ages of 30 and 60. In American women, however, the average age of menopause onset is 51. A woman must have missed a menstrual cycle for 12 months to be regarded as menopause. At this stage, the ovaries have completely stopped working and are no longer releasing eggs.

Hot flashes are the most common complaint among menopausal women. Furthermore, hot flashes may be accompanied by an increase in heart rate. As the pelvic floor relaxes, women may perceive less breast fullness, thinner hair, greater facial hair growth, or urine incontinence.

## POSTMENOPAUSE STAGE

A woman is termed postmenopausal when she has gone a complete year without a menstrual period and she will spend the remainder of her life at this stage. Fortunately, the symptoms that distinguish the perimenopause and menopausal years begin to fade at this time, leaving most women more physically comfortable. However, because estrogen levels are low, the risk of health issues such as osteoporosis and heart disease rises. A balanced lifestyle and hormone replacement medication can help women who have entered the postmenopausal period of life avoid hormone-related issues.

# SEVEN TIPS TO MAKE MENOPAUSE EASIER

### 1. Eat calcium and vitamin D foods.

Hormonal fluctuations during menopause might have an impact on your bones as it increases your chances of developing osteoporosis. It is essential to consume foods high in calcium and vitamin D to avoid this as both minerals are necessary for bone health. Vitamin D supplementation during menopause can reduce the incidence of fractures. Moreover, it is important to increase the consumption of dairy products such as milk, paneer, yogurt, and cheese. You should also eat more kale, collards, broccoli, spinach, tofu, and legumes, all of which are high in vitamin D.

### 2. Maintain healthy body weight.

Weight gain is natural during menopause. It could be caused by genetics, age, hormones, or a lifestyle change. During this time, women are more prone to gain belly fat and this may increase the risk of cardiovascular disease and diabetes. Weight gain during menopause can exacerbate the symptoms, so it is necessary to attempt to lose weight and maintain a healthy BMI.

### 3. Consume more fruits and vegetables.

A diet high in fruits and vegetables is the greatest approach to guarantee your body receives adequate nutrition. Fruits and vegetables are an excellent method to stay healthy while also losing weight. Overall, a diet high in fruits and vegetables can help you keep your bones healthy, maintain a healthy BMI, and avoid heart disease.

### 4. Avoid foods that may trigger menopausal symptoms.

Certain foods can cause menopausal symptoms which include night sweats, hot flashes, and mood swings. Alcohol, caffeine, and spicy foods are examples of these foods and the symptoms are worse when ingested at night. If you feel these symptoms after trying another meal, try eliminating it for a period and see if the symptoms improve.

### 5. Never skip meals.

It's not simply the foods you eat; it's the regularity of the meal. Eating regularly can help to keep menopausal symptoms under control. If you don't eat regularly, your symptoms are likely to worsen in addition to sabotaging your weight loss efforts, making things worse for you.

### 6. Consume extra protein.

With aging, you become more prone to lose lean muscle mass. To avoid this, it is important to consume more protein. Studies have shown that eating proteins throughout the day can help to reduce muscle loss caused by aging. This type of diet also promotes weight loss by keeping you fuller for longer periods and lowering your calorie intake. Overall, it assists you in losing weight over time.

### 7. Consume phytoestrogen-rich meals.

When we talk about phytoestrogens, we're talking about foods that mimic the actions of the female hormone estrogen which aids in hormone regulation. Tofu, tempeh, flaxseeds, sesame seeds, and beans are among these foods. It is therefore advisable to choose whole foods over supplements and manufactured phytoestrogen sources. A study found that a soy-rich diet reduced the intensity of night sweats and hot flashes in menopausal women or those approaching menopause.

# WHICH FOODS TO AVOID

Good nutrition can make a big change in how you feel with regard to menopause symptoms like mood swings, hot flashes, and exhaustion, as well as bloating and possible weight gain. As a woman going through menopause, there are certain foods you should learn to avoid. Some of them are:

- Spicy foods. Think twice before you add that hot sauce to your foods. Foods that rate high on the heat scale can trigger flushing, sweating and other symptoms of hot flashes. If you're looking to add a kick to your bland dish, it is advised that you use spices that bring as much flavor but without the heat such as cumin, turmeric and basil.

- Alcohol. Although it might not be necessary to swear off all cocktails and wine, there are plenty of good reasons to keep your alcohol consumption moderate. Some women have found that alcohol makes them more susceptible to hot flashes. Also, heavy drinking can increase one's risk to cardiovascular disease.

- Caffeine. Breaking away from that invigorating morning cup of pure energy will be difficult but you will have to do so. In its place, you could try green tea, peppermint tea and just generally stay away from all caffeinated drinks.

- Fatty foods. Steer clear of fast foods, fried foods and processed cakes, cookies and snacks. Try to keep your intake of fat-laden foods to a minimum except for fatty fish and nuts.

# HOW TO TREAT MENOPAUSE SYMPTOMS

Fortunately, many of the symptoms associated with menopause are temporary. You can take the following steps to help you reduce them or prevent their effects:

- **Get enough sleep**

Avoid caffeine, which can make it hard to get to sleep, and avoid drinking too much alcohol, which can interrupt sleep. Exercise during the day, although not right before bedtime. If hot flashes disturb your sleep, you may need to find a way to manage them before you can get adequate rest.

- **Eat a balanced diet**

Include a variety of fruits, vegetables and whole grains. Limit saturated fats, oils and sugars. Ask your doctor if you need calcium or vitamin D supplements to help meet daily requirements.

- **Exercise regularly**

Get regular physical activity or exercise on most days to help protect against heart disease, diabetes, osteoporosis and other conditions associated with aging.

- **Don't smoke**

Smoking increases your risk of heart disease, stroke, osteoporosis, cancer and a range of other health problems. It may also increase hot flashes and bring on earlier menopause.

- **Cool hot flashes**

Dress in layers, have a cold glass of water or go somewhere cooler. Try to pinpoint what triggers your hot flashes. For many women, triggers may include hot beverages, caffeine, spicy foods, alcohol, stress, hot weather and even a warm room.

- **Practice relaxation techniques**

Techniques such as deep breathing, paced breathing, guided imagery, massage and progressive muscle relaxation may help with menopausal symptoms. You can find a number of    books and online offerings that show different relaxation exercises.
These are just a few of the natural ways you can deal with the symptoms of menopause. Menopause requires no medical treatment. Any treatments administered by your doctor focus on relieving your symptoms and preventing or managing conditions that may be chronic as you continue to age. Treatments may include:

- **Low-dose antidepressants**

Certain antidepressants related to the class of drugs called selective serotonin reuptake inhibitors (SSRIs) may decrease menopausal hot flashes. A low-dose antidepressant for management of hot flashes may be useful for women who can't take estrogen for health reasons or for women who need an antidepressant for a mood disorder.

- **Clonidine**

Clonidine, a pill typically used to treat high blood pressure, might provide some relief from hot flashes.

- **Hormone therapy**

Estrogen therapy is the most effective treatment option for relieving menopausal hot flashes. Depending on your personal and family medical history, your doctor may recommend estrogen in the lowest dose and the shortest time frame needed to provide symptom relief for you. If you still have your uterus, you'll need progestin in addition to estrogen. Estrogen also helps prevent bone loss. Long-term use of hormone therapy may have some cardiovascular and breast cancer risks, but starting hormones around the time of menopause has shown benefits for some women. Talk to your doctor about the benefits and risks of hormone therapy and whether it's a safe choice for you.

- **Gabapentin**

Gabapentin is approved to treat seizures, but it has also been shown to help reduce hot flashes. This drug is useful in women who can't use estrogen therapy and in those who also have nighttime hot flashes.

These are just a few of the possible treatments your doctor could prescribe. Review your options yearly as your needs and treatment options may change.

| Day | Breakfast | AM Snack | Lunch | PM Snack | Dinner |
|---|---|---|---|---|---|
| DAY 1 | Orange-Cranberry Nut Muffins | 1 Apple | Garlic Butter Shrimp Quinoa | Poaches Pears and Green Tea | Broccoli Hash and with Poached Eggs |
| DAY 2 | Blueberry–Banana Oatmeal Bars | Sweet Potato Chips | Thai Coconut Curry Tofu | Handful Almonds | Kidney Bean Risotto |
| DAY 3 | Frozen Berry Yogurt | Handful Blueberries | Mashed Cod and Beans | Avocado Toast | Quinoa Salad |
| DAY 4 | Berry and Almond Overnight Oats | Green Smoothie with Cranberry | Risotto with Mushrooms | 1 Mango or Papaya | Tofu Stir Fry |
| DAY 5 | Orange and Banana Biscuits | 1 Pear | Vegan Parmesan Cauliflower Steaks over Hemp Pesto Zoodles | Exotic Dried Fruit Compote | Miso Soup with Veggies |
| DAY 6 | Scrambled Tofu | Beet Hummus | Tofu Stir Fry | Handful Blueberries | Shrimp and Quinoa Salad |
| DAY 7 | Green Smoothie | 1 Orange | Lemon, Olive, and Parsley Quinoa Cakes | Fruity Yogurt | Scrambled Tofu |
| DAY 8 | Oatmeal with Banana and Pollen | Peanut Butter Smoothie | Avocado Chickpeas Salad Collard Wraps | Handful Almonds | Sage Risotto |
| DAY 9 | Berry and Almond Overnight Oats | Green Smoothie with Cranberry | Garlic Butter Shrimp Quinoa | Poaches Pears and Green Tea | Broccoli Hash and with Poached Eggs |

| | | | | | |
|---|---|---|---|---|---|
| **DAY 10** | Scrambled Tofu | Beet Hummus | Thai Coconut Curry Tofu | Handful Almonds | Kidney Bean Risotto |
| **DAY 11** | Green Smoothie | 1 Orange | Mashed Cod and Beans | Avocado Toast | Quinoa Salad |
| **DAY 12** | Oatmeal with Banana and Pollen | Peanut Butter Smoothie | Tofu Stir Fry | Handful Blueberries | Shrimp and Quinoa Salad |
| **DAY 13** | Orange-Cranberry Nut Muffins | 1 Apple | Vegan Parmesan Cauliflower Steaks over Hemp Pesto Zoodles | Exotic Dried Fruit Compote | Miso Soup with Veggies |
| **DAY 14** | Blueberry–Banana Oatmeal Bars | Sweet Potato Chips | Tofu Stir Fry | Handful Blueberries | Shrimp and Quinoa Salad |
| **DAY 15** | Frozen Berry Yogurt | Handful Blueberries | Avocado Chickpeas Salad Collard Wraps | Handful Almonds | Sage Risotto |
| **DAY 16** | Berry and Almond Overnight Oats | Green Smoothie with Cranberry | Garlic Butter Shrimp Quinoa | Poaches Pears and Green Tea | Broccoli Hash and with Poached Eggs |
| **DAY 17** | Orange-Cranberry Nut Muffins | 1 Apple | Mashed Cod and Beans | Avocado Toast | Quinoa Salad |
| **DAY 18** | Blueberry–Banana Oatmeal Bars | Sweet Potato Chips | Thai Coconut Curry Tofu | Handful Almonds | Kidney Bean Risotto |

| | | | | | |
|---|---|---|---|---|---|
| **DAY 19** | Scrambled Tofu | Beet Hummus | Vegan Parmesan Cauliflower Steaks over Hemp Pesto Zoodles | Exotic Dried Fruit Compote | Miso Soup with Veggies |
| **DAY 20** | Green Smoothie | 1 Orange | Mashed Cod and Beans | Avocado Toast | Quinoa Salad |
| **DAY 21** | Oatmeal with Banana and Pollen | Peanut Butter Smoothie | Lemon, Olive, and Parsley Quinoa Cakes | Fruity Yogurt | Scrambled Tofu |

# 1. Orange-Cranberry Nut Muffins

Time: 30 minutes

Calories: 221g|Carbohydrate: 35 grams |fat: 9 grams |Protein: 4 grams

## Ingredients:

- 125g all-purpose flour
- 30g unprocessed bran and 90g whole wheat flour
- 5g of topping and 100g of of sugar (optional)
- 12g of baking soda
- 20g Baking powder
- Salt, 2g
- 100g of cranberries, dried
- 50g chopped walnuts

- 50g Buttermilk
- 700ml of vegetable oil
- 1 big egg
- 1 orange zest
- 4.5 ml of orange flavoring
- 1g of ground cinnamon and 4.5ml of vanilla extract (optional)

## Directions:

1. Turn on the oven's dial to 191°C. Use paper liners to line a standard muffin pan.
2. Combine the flours, bran, sugar, baking soda, baking powder, salt, walnuts, and cranberries in a large bowl.
3. Combine the buttermilk, oil, egg, orange zest, orange extract, and vanilla in a medium basin.
4. Combine the flour mixture with the buttermilk mixture by stirring only until mixed. Avoid overmixing. Fill each muffin cup with an even amount of the batter. Sprinkle a little of the mixture on top of each muffin, if preferred, by combining sugar and the cinnamon in a small bowl.
5. When a toothpick is inserted in the center of a muffin, it should come out clean after 16 to 18 minutes of baking. Before eating, place on a wire rack to cool for 15 minutes.

# 2. Blueberry–Banana Oatmeal Bars

Time: 40 minutes

Calories: 194g |Carbohydrate: 28 grams |fat: 7 grams |Protein: 5 grams

## Ingredients:

- ❖ 600g of oats
- ❖ Salt
- ❖ 10g baking powder
- ❖ 2g of ground cinnamon (optional)
- ❖ 3 ripe medium bananas, mashed well

- ❖ 70ml of canola oil
- ❖ 2 large eggs
- ❖ 4.5ml of vanilla extract
- ❖ 450ml 1% low-fat milk
- ❖ 350g of frozen fresh blueberries

## Directions:

1. Set the oven to 177°C for starters. Spray cooking spray in a 9 by 11-inch baking pan.
2. Combine the oats, salt, baking powder, and cinnamon, if using, in a sizable basin. Whisk the mashed bananas, oil, eggs, and vanilla until thoroughly blended and set aside in a separate big dish. Milk is whisked in.
3. Mix the oat mixture with the banana mixture. To blend, thoroughly stir. Add the blueberries slowly. It will be soupy batter. Place the baking pan with the batter inside.
4. Bake until firm, about 25 to 30 minutes. After taking it out of the oven, let it cool for 15 minutes on a wire rack. Cut into 12 pieces of the same size. Place in an airtight jar and keep in the refrigerator if you want to enjoy it later.

# 3. Waldorf Salad

Time: 15 minutes

Calories: 242.5 kCal |Protein: 2 grams |Fat: 20.8 grams |Carbohydrate: 24.grams

## Ingredients:

- ❖ 30g of pecans
- ❖ 4 apples, such as Cortland, Empire, or Red Delicious
- ❖ Lemon juice (freshly squeezed)
- ❖ 4 celery stalks, thinly sliced
- ❖ 30g of halved red seedless grapes
- ❖ 50ml of plain yogurt
- ❖ 600g of arugula

## Directions:

1. Toast the pecans in a skillet for a few minutes to bring out their flavor. When they are cool enough to handle, coarsely chop them.
2. Peel and chop the apples, then toss them in a bowl with the lemon juice to prevent them from discoloring.
3. Mix well the apples with the celery, grapes, and half of the pecans. Stir in the yogurt and then gently toss together.
4. Divide the arugula among four serving plates and spoon over the salad mixture. Sprinkle the remaining nuts over the salad.

# 4. Exotic Dried Fruit Compote

Time: 15 minutes

Calories: 36 kCal |Fat: 0.07 grams |Carbohydrates: 9.28 grams |Protein: 0.38 grams

## Ingredients:
- 30g of dried peaches
- 30g of dried apricots
- 40g of dried pineapple chunks
- 30g of dried mango slices
- 150ml unsweetened apple juice
- 150ml of plain yogurt (optional)

## Directions:
1. Combine the apple juice and dried fruit in a small saucepan. Bring the mixture slowly to a boil, then lower the heat, cover it, and simmer for 10 minutes.
2. Spoon into serving bowls and, if using, sprinkle a spoonful of yoghurt on top of each portion. Serve right away.

# 5. Frozen Berry Yogurt

Time: 20 minutes

Calories: 60 |Fat: 0.5 grams |Carbohydrates: 15 grams |Protein: 1 gram

## Ingredients:
- 100g raspberries
- 100g blackberries
- 100g strawberries
- 1 extra-large egg

- 75ml Greek-style yogurt
- 100ml of red wine
- 5g powdered gelatin
- fresh berries, to decorate

## Directions:
1. Blend the strawberries, blackberries, and raspberries in a food processor until they are completely smooth. Push the puree through a strainer into a basin to catch the seeds.
2. Break one egg, then divide the white and yolk into two bowls. Egg white should be kept aside as you combine the egg yolk and yoghurt with the fruit puree.
3. Pour the wine into a heat-resistant bowl and top with the gelatin. Set the bowl over a pot of simmering water for 5 minutes to soften the gelatin, then leave it there until it dissolves. While continuously beating, stream a steady stream of the mixture into the fruit puree. Put the mixture in a freezer and let it sit there for two hours, or until it becomes slushy.
4. In a pristine, grease-free basin, beat the egg white until it is extremely firm. Fold the egg white into the berry mixture after removing it from the freezer. Go back to the freezer and keep it there for 2 more hours. Scoop the berry yoghurt ice into serving bowls, then top with your preferred fresh berries to serve.

# 6. Orange and Banana Biscuits

Time: 25 minutes

Calories:260 |Carbohydrates: 18 grams |Fat: 1 gram |Protein: 0 grams

## Ingredients:

- sunflower oil, for oiling
- 75g white all-purpose our, plus extra for dusting, and for rolling, if needed
- 150g whole-wheat our
- 10g baking powder
- 1g ground cinnamon
- 20g unsalted butter, diced and chilled
- 30g demerara sugar or other raw sugar
- 60ml of milk, plus extra for brushing
- 1 ripe banana, peeled and mashed
- Finely grated rind of 1 orange
- Fresh raspberries, lightly mashed

## Directions:

1. Preheat the oven to 200°C. Lightly oil a baking sheet.
2. In a large basin, combine the flour, baking soda, and cinnamon. Add the butter and stir with your hands until the mixture resembles coarse bread crumbs. Add the sugar and stir. In the center of the dry ingredients, create a well, and add the milk. Mix in the orange rind and mashed banana to create a soft dough. The dough will be extremely moist.
3. Roll out the dough to a thickness of 1/4 inch after turning it out onto a lightly oared surface. Cut out 12 biscuits with a 212-inch cookie cutter, rerolling any scraps of dough as needed, and set them on the prepared baking pan. Bake for 10–12 minutes in a preheated oven after brushing with milk.
4. After taking the biscuits out of the oven, cut them in half and top with the raspberries.

# 7. Chicken Avocado Salad

Time: 20 minutes

Calories: 373.6 |Fat: 19.8 grams |Carbohydrate: 8.8 grams |Protein: 40.8 grams

## Ingredients:

- 500g of mixed salad greens, including radicchio, endive, and beet leaves
- 300g of cooked, skinless, and boneless chicken shreds
- two satsumas divided into segments.
- 12 red onions, halved, and thinly sliced 2 celery stalks
- fresh chives, finely chopped
- two avocadoes
- To garnish, use toasted sunflower seeds.
- serving of whole-wheat pita bread

## Directions:

1. Add roughly a third of the dressing to the salad leaves in a bowl and gently toss. Toss once more after adding the chicken, satsumas, celery, onion, chives, and remaining dressing.
2. Halve the avocados, remove the pit, and then peel the skin. To prevent the avocado slices from turning brown, slice them into thin slices, add it to the other ingredients, and gently toss everything together.
3. Arrange on serving plates, sprinkle sun over seeds over the top, and serve immediately with whole-wheat pita bread.

# 8. Cherry Yogurt Sundae

Time: 15 minutes

Calories: 215 |Fat: 2 grams |Carbohydrate: 48 grams |Protein: 4 grams

## Ingredients:

- 125g of strawberry hulls
- Honey
- 15 milliliters of vanilla bean paste or extract
- 120 ml of active cultures in plain yoghurt
- 125g of pitted, halved, fresh cherries
- 40g of hazelnuts, roughly chopped

## Directions:

1. Blend the strawberries until they are smooth in a blender. Place in a bowl and combine with the honey and vanilla bean paste. The yoghurt should be lightly incorporated with the strawberry-vanilla sauce.
2. Place the cherries in two plates and top with the strawberry yoghurt mixture. Prior to serving, top them with the hazelnuts.

# 9. Peanut Butter Smoothie

Time: 5 minutes

394 calories |carbohydrates**.**42 grammes |Fat: 18 grammes |protein. 23 grammes

## Ingredients:
- ❖ 65ml of plain fat-free Greek yogurt
- ❖ 30ml 1% low-fat milk
- ❖ 10g natural peanut butter (without added sugar, if desired)
- ❖ 1 frozen medium banana
- ❖ Vanilla extract

## Directions:
1. Place all the ingredients in a blender and blend on high speed for 45 seconds or until smooth.
2. This creamy beverage contains peanut butter, which promotes heart health. For a meal, serve this comforting beverage with some whole-wheat toast.

# 10. Berry and Almond Overnight Oats
Time: 15 minutes

Calories: 299 | Carbohydrate: 44 grams | Fat: 7 grams | Protein: 17 grams

**Ingredients:**
- ❖ 70g of quick or old-fashioned rolled oats
- ❖ 60ml 1% low-fat milk
- ❖ 40ml plain fat-free Greek yogurt
- ❖ Sweetener of choice, as desired
- ❖ 50g of fresh raspberries, sliced strawberries, blackberries, or blueberries, or a combination
- ❖ 5g of sliced almonds

**Directions:**
1. Combine the oats, milk, yogurt, and sweetener in a container with a lid, such as a mason jar. Shake or stir until well combined. Refrigerate overnight. Add the fruit and almonds just before eating.
2. A modest food with powerful properties, oats can reduce blood cholesterol and the risk of heart disease. When you don't have time to cook breakfast in the morning, these overnight oats with crunchy sliced almonds and delicious berries are a welcome sight!

# 11. Avocado Toast

Time: 10 minutes

## COTTAGE CHEESE AND AVOCADO WERE USED IN THE PREP:
## COTTAGE CHEESE:

calories. 131 |carbohydrates. 17 grammes |Fat: 2 grammes | Protein. 4grammes

## AVOCADO AND EGGS:

calories. 168 |carbohydrates. 16 grammes |Fat 7 grammes |protein 11grammes

## Ingredients:

- ❖ 1 egg, fried over easy or scrambled, or 60g of low-fat cottage cheese
- ❖ Whole-grain bread slice weighing 28 grammes, with a pitted and sliced half of an avocado.
- ❖ Freshly ground black pepper and salt (optional)

## Directions:

1. Add the cottage cheese to a blender, and process for about 45 seconds, or until smooth.
2. Cover the toast with cottage cheese. Add the avocado and salt & pepper to taste on top. Alternately, spread the cooked egg and avocado on the toast.

# 12. Cranberry and Orange Smoothie

Time: 5 minutes

Calories: 190 grams |fat: 3.9 grams |Carbohydrates: 27 grams |Protein: 11 grams

**Ingredients:**

- ❖ 1 orange
- ❖ Cranberries
- ❖ 1 banana
- ❖ Plain yogurt
- ❖ Fine shreds of orange zest, to decorate

**Directions:**

1. Peel the orange, but keep a little of the white pith.
2. In a blender, mix the orange and cranberries until they are completely smooth. Yogurt and the peeled banana should be added before blending.
3. Pour into glasses, top with orange zest slivers, and serve.

# 13. Fig and Watermelon Salad

Time: 15 minutes

Calories: 147 grams |Fat: 5.7 grams |Carbohydrates: 23 grams |Protein: 2 grams

## Ingredients:

- ❖ 1 watermelon (about 1.5 kg)
- ❖ 4 figs and 4 seedless red grapes

### Dressing:

- ❖ Lime rind, grated
- ❖ 1 orange's grated rind and juice
- ❖ Maple syrup
- ❖ Honey

## Directions:

1. Quarter the watermelon, then remove and discard the seeds. Remove the esh from the rind by cutting it, then cut it into 1-inch cubes. Put the grapes and watermelon cubes in a basin. Add to the bowl after cutting each g lengthwise into 8 wedges.
2. In a small saucepan, combine the lime rind, orange rind and juice, maple syrup, and honey to make the dressing. Using low heat, bring to a boil. Stir after pouring the mixture over the fruit. Cool down. Stir once more, cover, and chill for at least one hour in the refrigerator.
3. Evenly distribute the fruit salad among the four serving bowls and then serve.

# 14. Beet Hummus

Time: 1 hour 15 minutes

Calories: 491 grams |Fat: 39 grams |Carbohydrates: 27 grams |Protein: 12 grams

## Ingredients:

- ❖ 425 grammes of washed and drained canned chickpeas
- ❖ 1 clove of chopped garlic,
- ❖ 2 prepared beets
- ❖ Tahini
- ❖ Olive oil and half a squeezed lemon
- ❖ Pepper and salt
- ❖ Cherry tomatoes and vegetable sticks will be served.

## Directions:

1. Blend the chickpeas, garlic, and beets in a food processor until the mixture resembles coarse crumbs.
2. Once the hummus has reached the desired consistency, add the tahini, lemon juice, and olive oil and pulse once more. Add salt and pepper to taste.
3. Dish the hummus with cherry tomatoes and vegetable sticks.

# 15. Asparagus with Poached Eggs and Parmesan

## Time: 30 minutes

Calories: 260 grams |Fat: 22 grams |Carbohydrates: 7 grams |Protein: 10 grams

## Ingredients:

- ❖ 20 trimmed asparagus spears, weighing around 340 grammes
- ❖ Four big eggs
- ❖ Parmesan cheese shavings

## Directions:

1. Bring water in two saucepans to a boil. In one pan, add the asparagus, bring back to a simmer, and cook for 5 minutes, or until asparagus is just tender.
2. In the meantime, turn the heat down to a simmer in the second saucepan and carefully crack each egg in one at a time. If the whites are barely set but the yolks are still mushy, poach the eggs for three minutes. Once finished, remove.
3. Drain the asparagus, then distribute it among four dishes for serving. Add an egg and some Parmesan cheese to the top of each asparagus platter. You may now serve it.

# 16. Tofu and Bok Choy Stir-fry

Time: 20 minutes

Calories: 560 grams |Fat: 25 grams |Carbohydrates: 66 grams |Protein: 27 grams

**Ingredients:**
- ❖ Olive oil or sunflower oil
- ❖ Finely chopped bok choy
- ❖ Drained and diced tofu
- ❖ 1 sliced garlic clove
- ❖ Sweet chili sauce
- ❖ Light soy sauce

**Directions:**
1. Add the tofu in batches and stir-fry for 2-3 minutes, or until brown, in a wok with heated oil. Take out and place aside.
2. Stir-fry the bok choy for a few seconds, until it is soft and wilted. Take out of the wok and place aside
3. Stir-fry the garlic for 30 seconds after adding the remaining oil to the wok. Bring to a boil after adding the soy sauce and chili sauce.
4. Toss the tofu and bok choy gently in the skillet to coat with the sauce. Serve right away.

# 17. Gazpacho with Celery Salsa
Time: 30 minutes

Calories: 139 kcal |Fat: 9 grams |Carbohydrates: 15 grams |Protein: 3 grams

## Ingredients:
- ❖ 2 thick slices day-old fresh white bread, crusts removed
- ❖ 60ml of water, for soaking
- ❖ 4 tomatoes, seeded and skinned
- ❖ 1 small cucumber, peeled, seeded, and chopped
- ❖ 1 large red chili, seeded and chopped
- ❖ 1 large garlic clove
- ❖ Olive oil
- ❖ Lemon juice freshly squeezed

## Celery salsa
- ❖ 1 celery stalk, sliced
- ❖ 1 small avocado, skinned, pitted, and diced
- ❖ 6 large basil leaves

## Directions:
1. Soak one of the bread slices for five minutes in the water.
2. In a blender, add the bread, tomatoes, cucumber, garlic, oil, lemon juice (reserved), and the remaining 3/4 of the chili. Blend until blended but still a bit chunky. Give it two to three hours to chill.
3. Prepare the celery salsa just before serving. Combine the celery, avocado, basil, remaining chili, lemon juice that has been set aside, and those ingredients in a bowl.
4. Cube the remaining piece of bread. The bread should be browned and crisp for about 5 minutes in a skillet with the remaining olive oil.
5. Place a generous spoonful of the salsa and some croutons on top of each serving bowl after ladling the soup into them.

# 18. Sautéed Brussels Sprouts

Time: 20 minutes

Calories: 114 kcal |Fat: 7 grams |Carbohydrates: 11 grams |Protein: 4 grams

## Ingredients:

- Olive oil
- 1 pound of brussels sprouts, split in half lengthwise
- 2 pieces of unsmoked bacon,
- Chopped, 4 shallots, 60ml of vegetable stock, and the juice from half a lemon
- To serve, 40g of Parmesan cheese shavings

## Directions:

1. In a large skillet set over medium heat, add the olive oil and cook the bacon for two to three minutes.
2. Place the sprouts on top, cut-side down, and top with the shallots. After about 5 minutes, flip the sprouts over and cook them for an additional 5 minutes on the other side.
3. Pour the vegetable stock over the sprouts and steam-fry for a few minutes, or until the sprouts are tender and the liquid has been absorbed.
4. Add some lemon juice, then serve right away with some Parmesan cheese shavings.

# 19. Mixed Cabbage Coleslaw

Time: 5 minutes

Calories: 52.2 grams |Fat: 1.8 grams |Carbohydrates: 8.6 grams |Protein: 1.2 grams

## Ingredients:
- ❖ shredded red cabbage, fine
- ❖ shreds of white cabbage, finely (or green cabbage if white cabbage is not available)
- ❖ shredded green cabbage, fine
- ❖ two shredded carrots and one thinly sliced white onion

- ❖ 2 chopped red apples
- ❖ 60 ml orange juice
- ❖ 2 cut celery stalks
- ❖ corn kernels in a can
- ❖ 20g of raisins

## Dressing
- ❖ 40ml low-fat plain yogurt

- ❖ Freshly chopped parsley

## Directions:
1. Add the carrots and onion to the cabbages in a bowl. Add the apples, any leftover orange juice, the celery, corn, and raisins to the cabbages after tossing them in the orange juice. Mix well.
2. Combine the yoghurt and parsley in a bowl to make the dressing, then drizzle it over the cabbage mixture. Stir, then plate.

# 20. Zucchini, Carrot, and Tomato Frittata

Time: 35 minutes

Calories: 259.9 kcal |Fat: 28.88 grams |Carbohydrates: 20.16 grams |Protein: 12.69 grams

## Ingredients:

- ❖ Olive oil
- ❖ 1 onion, peeled and cut into wedges
- ❖ 1-2 smashed garlic cloves
- ❖ 2 eggs
- ❖ Two egg whites.
- ❖ Shredded zucchini, two carrots, two tomatoes, and fresh basil for garnish.

## Directions:

1. In a sizable nonstick skillet, heat the olive oil over medium heat. Add the onion and garlic, and cook, turning often, for 5 minutes. The eggs and egg whites should be combined in a bowl before being added to the skillet. Pull the egg mixture from the sides of the skillet toward the centre using a spatula or fork, allowing the raw egg to take its place.
2. After the bottom has barely set, add the tomatoes, zucchini, and carrots. The eggs should continue to cook at a low temperature until they are cooked to your liking.
3. Place on plates for serving. Slice the frittata into quarters, garnish with the basil slivers, and serve warm or cold.

# 21. Baked Sweet Potatoes with Hummus

Time: 30 minutes

Calories: 142 grams |Fat: 0.2 grams |Carbohydrates: 32.7 grams |Protein: 3.2 grams

## Ingredients:

- ❖ 6 unpeeled sweet potatoes
- ❖ Almond oil
- ❖ Table salt
- ❖ Fresh at-leaf parsley, chopped, served with salad greens
- ❖ 425 grammes of can of rinsed and drained chickpeas
- ❖ Two lemons' juice
- ❖ Tahini
- ❖ Olive oil
- ❖ 1 smashed garlic clove

## Directions:

1. Set the oven's temperature to 218°C. The sweet potatoes should be pierced all over with a fork before being rubbed with olive oil and salt. Roast the sweet potatoes for 35 to 45 minutes, or until a knife inserted into one of them comes out clean.
2. Blend the chickpeas with a few spoons of lemon juice until a thick puree is produced. Process one again after including the tahini, olive oil, and garlic. Salt the food before reprocessing. If desired, taste and add more lemon juice. Scrape into a bowl, wrap in plastic wrap, and place in the refrigerator until needed.
3. Slit each potato lengthwise and squeeze it open once it is ready. Serve with some salad leaves and parsley as a garnish.

# 22. Stir-fried Bean Sprouts

Time: 50 minutes

Calories: 70 kcal |Fat: 4 grams |Carbohydrates: 8 grams |Protein: 4 grams

## Ingredients:
- Olive or peanut oil
- Bean sprouts
- Finely chopped scallion
- Salt
- 30g of sugar

## Directions:
1. Heat the oil in a deep skillet or wok over high heat, then stir-fry the bean sprouts and scallion for about a minute. Stir in the sugar and salt.
2. Turn off the heat and serve.

# 23. Cauliflower and Beans with cashew Nuts

Time: 1 hour

Calories: 345 kcal |Fat: 15 grams |Carbohydrates: 47 grams |Protein: 12 grams

## Ingredients:

- Vegetable or peanut oil
- Spice oil
- One sliced onion
- Two minced garlic cloves for the Thai red curry paste
- 1 little head of cauliflower that has been chopped into florets
- 3-5-inch lengths of green beans
- 70ml of a vegetable stock
- Chinese soy sauce
- To garnish, toast some cashew nuts.

## Directions:

1. In a wok that has been heated with both oils, stir-fry the onion and garlic until they are tender. Stir-fry the curry paste for a few minutes after adding it.
2. Stir-fry the beans and cauliflower for 3 to 4 minutes, or until they are tender. Add the stock and soy sauce, then boil for a couple of minutes. Serve right away with cashew nut garnish.

# 24. Fennel and Tomato Soup with Shrimp
Time: 1 hour

Calories: 115 kcal |Fat: 7 grams |Carbohydrates: 10 grams |Protein: 3 grams

## Ingredients:
- Olive oil
- 1 large onion, halved and sliced
- 2 large fennel bulbs, halved and sliced
- 1 small potato, peeled and diced
- 700ml of water
- 300ml of tomato juice, plus extra if needed
- 1 bay leaf
- 400g cooked, peeled small shrimp
- 2 tomatoes, skinned, seeded, and chopped
- Snipped fresh dill
- Salt and pepper
- Dill sprigs, to garnish

## Directions:
1. In a big pot set over medium heat, warm the olive oil. When the onion is barely softened, add the fennel and onion, and simmer for 3 to 4 minutes, turning regularly.
2. Include the bay leaf, potato, water, tomato juice, and salt to taste. When the vegetables are tender, reduce the heat, cover the pan, and simmer for about 25 minutes, stirring occasionally.
3. Take out and throw away the bay leaf after letting the soup cool slightly. Transfer to a blender and blend until smooth, if required blending in batches. (If using a blender, remove and set aside the cooking liquid. The soup solids should be pureed with just enough cooking liquid to moisten them, then combined with the liquid that was set aside.
4. Add the shrimp and put the soup back in the pot. To reheat the soup and let it take on the taste of the shrimp, simmer it gently for about 10 minutes.
5. Add the dill and tomatoes after that. To taste and season as necessary. If needed, add a bit extra tomato liquid to thin the soup. Serve immediately after ladling into serving bowls and adding dill sprigs as a garnish.

# 25. Lemon and Garlic Spinach
Time: 15 minutes

Calories: 80 kcal |Fat: 4 grams |Carbohydrates: 0 grams | Protein. 0gram

## Ingredients:
- ❖ Almond oil
- ❖ 450 grammes of torn or shredded spinach
- ❖ 2 thinly sliced garlic cloves, and lemon juice

## Directions:
1. In a big skillet over high heat, heat the olive oil. When the spinach is tender, continue cooking while tossing in the garlic. Take care not to let the spinach burn.
2. Take the dish from the fire, transfer it to a serving bowl, and squeeze some lemon juice over it. Mix thoroughly and serve warm or at room temperature.

# 26. Peas with Lettuce, Shallots, and Mint

Time: 20 minutes

Calories: 105 kcal | Fat: 6 grams |Carbohydrates: 8 grams |Protein: 5 grams

## Ingredients:
- ❖ Fresh peas with shells
- ❖ 8 romaine lettuce leaves, shredded
- ❖ 2 shallots, thinly sliced
- ❖ 1 garlic clove, finely diced
- ❖ 3 fresh mint sprigs, plus more for garnish.
- ❖ Butter, sugar, or vegetable oil
- ❖ Pepper and salt

## Directions:
1. Bring water in a pot to a boil. Wax paper that has been dampened should be used to line a steamer.
2. Place the mint sprigs, lettuce, shallots, and garlic in the steamer with the peas. Add some sugar and butter, then sprinkle. Add salt and pepper to taste.
3. Place the steamer over the pan of boiling water and cover it with a tight-fitting lid. The peas should steam for about 4 minutes or until they are soft.
4. Cut the mint sprigs off and throw them away. Place the vegetables in a serving dish, top with a sprig of fresh mint, and serve right away.

# 27. Broccoli Hash with Poached Eggs
Time: 10 minutes

Calories: 385 kcal |Fat: 17 grams |Carbohydrates: 31 grams |Protein: 22 grams

## Ingredients:
- four potatoes
- 2 inch squares
- Orets, little broccoli, sunflower oil
- A large red bell pepper that has been seeded and finely diced, along with one onion, pulverised
- red Pepper
- Four big eggs
- Pepper and salt

## Directions:
1. Boil the potatoes for 6 minutes in lightly salted water. Good drainage Broccoli should be steamed or blanched for 3 minutes.
2. Add the onion and red bell pepper to a big skillet with the oil already heated over high heat, and cook for a couple of minutes to soften. When the potatoes are cooked, add them and simmer them for 6 to 8 minutes, occasionally tossing. Broccoli and crushed red pepper are added, and the mixture is cooked over low heat, occasionally being turned, until golden brown. Add salt and pepper to taste.
3. In the meantime, heat a sizable pot of water to just below simmering. The eggs should be gently poached for 3 to 4 minutes, or until softly set.
4. Place the hash on serving plates, then place an egg on top of each serving.

# 28. Chicken and Pine Nuts with Couscous

Time: 1 hour 20 minutes

Calories: 348 kcal | Fat: 20 grams |Carbohydrates: 16 grams |Protein: 26.3 grams

## Ingredients:
- 1-2 strands of saffron
- Golden raisins with couscous
- Heating up chicken or veggie stock to a boil
- 8 strips from one chicken breastlet, weighing approximately 120 grammes.
- Corn grain
- Aspen nuts
- Ten cherry tomatoes, quartered
- Chopped scallions, two
- To garnish, use fresh cilantro leaves.

## Dressing
- Neatly chopped fresh cilantro leaves
- Juice from half a lemon
- Olive oil

## Directions:
1. Add the hot stock to the heatproof dish with the saffron, couscous, and golden raisins. 15 minutes should pass after a single stir.
2. In the meantime, combine the dressing's components.
3. For about 4 minutes, brown the chicken strips on all sides in a hot, nonstick skillet. After turning the heat down to medium, add the corn and pine nuts, and simmer for an additional two minutes while stirring occasionally. The chicken should be taken out of the skillet and put aside.
4. Toss the couscous in the skillet with the tomatoes, dressing, and scallions after fluffing it up with a fork. Stirring gently, heat for 1 minute, or until thoroughly warmed.
5. Spoon onto a serving plate, top with chicken pieces, and add cilantro leaves as a garnish.

# 29. Pork with Cinammon

Time: 50 minutes

Calories: 414 grams | Fat: 25.5 grams Carbohydrates: 0 grams |Protein: 43.7 grams

## Ingredients:

- ❖ Pork tenderloin, diced, 450 grammes
- ❖ Vegetable oil
- ❖ 1 large onion, cut; 2 inches of freshly chopped ginger;
- ❖ 4 freshly minced garlic cloves

- ❖ 1-stick of cinnamon
- ❖ 6 pods of green cardamom
- ❖ 6 complete cloves
- ❖ 1 bay leaf,
- ❖ Water
- ❖ Salt

## Marinade

- ❖ Coarse coriander
- ❖ Cumin seed powder

- ❖ Chili powder
- ❖ Plain yoghurt

## Directions:

1. In a small dish, combine the yoghurt, coriander, cumin, and chilli powder to make the marinade. Put the marinade and the meat in a sizable, shallow nonmetallic dish and turn to coat well. For 30 minutes, marinate in the refrigerator with a cover made of plastic wrap.
2. In a sizable, heavy saucepan, heat the oil. The onion should be softened after 5 minutes of low heat cooking with intermittent tossing. Add the bay leaves, ginger, garlic, cinnamon stick, cardamom pods, and other spices; simmer for two minutes, stirring constantly, or until the spices begin to smell. Salt the mixture after adding the meat, water, and marinade. Boil for 30 minutes, then turn down the heat, cover, and simmer. Take out and throw away the bay leaves.
3. Transfer the meat mixture to a wok or a sizable, heavy skillet that has been prepared. Cook the meat mixture over low heat, stirring frequently, until it is dry and tender. If necessary, add a little water every now and again to keep it from sticking to the wok. Serve right away.

# 30. Turkey Kabobs with Cilantro Pesto

Time: 45 minutes

Calories: 563 kcal | Fat: 34 grams | Carbohydrates: 12 grams | Protein: 51 grams

## Ingredients:

- 4 turkey steaks, about 100g each, cut into 2-inch cubes
- 2 zucchinis, thickly sliced
- 1 red and 1 yellow bell pepper, seeded and cut into 2-inch cubes
- 8 cherry tomatoes
- 8 pearl onions, peeled

## Marinade

- 75ml of olive oil
- 40ml of dry white wine
- 10g of green peppercorns, crushed
- 25g of chopped fresh cilantro
- Salt

## Cilantro pesto

- 200g of fresh cilantro leaves
- 150g of fresh parsley leaves
- 1 garlic clove
- 100g pine nuts
- 100g grated parmesan cheese
- 150g extra virgin olive oil
- Lemon juice

## Directions:

1. Firstly, put the turkey in a big glass bowl. Combine the olive oil, wine, peppercorns, cilantro, and salt in a small bowl to make the marinade. When the turkey is completely covered, pour the mixture over it and toss. For two hours, marinate in the refrigerator with a cover made of plastic.
2. Place the cilantro and parsley in a blender and process until finely chopped to create the cilantro pesto. Process the garlic and pine nuts after adding them. Olive oil, lemon juice, and Parmesan cheese are added; process just long enough to combine. When ready, transfer to a bowl, cover, and chill in the fridge.
3. To avoid burning, soak wooden skewers in water for 30 minutes before using them. Set a broiler to medium-high heat. Drain the turkey and keep the marinade aside. 8 metal or pre-soaked wooden skewers should be used to alternately thread the turkey, zucchini slices, bell pepper pieces, tomatoes, and onions. Cook under the preheated broiler for 10 minutes, or until well cooked, turning frequently and sprinkling with the marinade. Serve right away with the pesto made from cilantro.

# 31. Roasted Salmon with Lemon and Herbs

Time: 30 minutes

Calories: 397 kcal |Fat: 27 grams |Carbohydrates: 1 gram |Protein: 35 grams

**Ingredients:**

- 75ml of virgin olive oil
- 1 onion, sliced
- 1 leek, sliced
- Juice from half a lemon
- 25g of chopped fresh parsley
- 25g of chopped fresh dill
- 450g of salmon llets
- Salt and pepper
- Freshly cooked baby spinach leaves and lemon wedges, to serve

**Directions:**

1. Set the oven to 205°C for starters. Over medium heat, warm up the oil in a skillet. For about 4 minutes, while stirring, sauté the onion and leek until they are just beginning to soften.
2. In the meantime, combine the remaining oil, lemon juice, and herbs in a small bowl. Add salt and pepper to taste. Ensure thorough mixing. The fish should be washed in cold running water and then dried with paper towels. Sh should be arranged in a small, oven-safe baking dish.
3. Spread the onion across the skillet after turning off the heat. Make sure everything is completely covered by the oil mixture before pouring it over the top. For about 10 minutes, or until the meat is thoroughly cooked, roast in the center of the preheated oven.
4. Place the cooked spinach on plates for dishing. Place the fish and vegetables on top of the spinach after they have been taken out of the oven. Serve right away with lemon slices on the side.

# 32. Beans and Artichokes with Seared Tuna

Time: 15 minutes

Calories: 463 kcal |Fat: 29 grams |Carbohydrates: 30 grams |Protein: 15 grams

## Ingredients:
- 190ml of extra virgin olive oil
- Juice from a lemon
- 2g of crushed red pepper
- 4 thin fresh tuna steaks, about a 100g each
- 250g of dried cannellini beans, soaked overnight
- 1 shallot, finely chopped
- 1 garlic clove, crushed
- 10g of finely chopped rosemary
- 25g of chopped at-leaf parsley
- 4 oil-cured artichokes, quartered
- 4 vine-ripened tomatoes, sliced lengthwise into segments
- 16 ripe black olives, pitted
- Salt and pepper
- Lemon wedges, to serve

## Directions:
1. Combine the lemon juice, pepper, crushed red pepper, and olive oil in a shallow dish. Add the tuna steaks and flip them occasionally for an hour at room temperature.
2. In the meantime, rinse the beans and add enough fresh water to cover in a pot. Bring to a boil before quickly boiling for 15 minutes. Cook for an additional 30 minutes, with the heat slightly reduced, or until the food is cooked but not falling apart. During the final five minutes of cooking, add salt.
3. Transfer the rinsed beans to a basin. Stir in the shallot, garlic, rosemary, parsley, and remaining lemon juice while the food is still warm. Toss with the olive oil. Add salt and pepper to taste. Let the flavors mingle for at least 30 minutes before serving.
4. In a saucepan, heat the olive oil until it is hot. Over high heat, add the tuna and the marinade, and sear for one to two minutes on each side. Remove from the pan and allow to slightly cool.
5. Place the beans on a serving platter. Add the artichokes, tomatoes, and olives after seasoning with additional oil as needed. Tuna should be flaked and arranged on top. With lemon wedges for squeezing over, serve right away.

# 33. Broiled Sardines with Mediterranean Spinach

Time: 45 minutes

Calories: 536 kcal |Fat: 14 grams |Carbohydrates: 75 grams |Protein: 25 grams

## Ingredients:
- 70ml of olive oil, plus extra for brushing and oiling
- Finely grated rind and juice of 1 orange
- 1 small red onion, thinly sliced
- 1 garlic clove, nely chopped
- 1 small red chile, seeded and nely chopped, or pinch of crushed red pepper
- 12 sprigs fresh thyme
- 12 sardines, heads removed, gutted, and rinsed inside and out

## Mediterranean spinach
- 20ml of olive oil
- 1 onion, chopped
- 1 large garlic clove
- 6g of ground coriander
- 6g of ground cumin
- 900g of spinach leaves
- 150g of pine nuts, lightly toasted
- Salt and pepper

## Directions:
1. In a flat bowl big enough to hold all the sardines, combine the olive oil, orange rind and juice, onion, garlic, and chile. Beat until well combined. Add the fish to the marinade, then use your hands to coat it. Place a thyme sprig into each sardine.
2. In a skillet over medium-high heat, warm the oil to prepare the Mediterranean spinach. Crush the garlic, add it to the skillet, and cook the onion for a further three minutes while stirring. At this point, the onion should be tender. Add a bit of salt and the coriander and cumin, and simmer for another minute while stirring. Using a wooden spoon, put the spinach into the skillet so that it contains just the water that is still on its leaves. Add salt and pepper to taste. Cook for 8 minutes while stirring frequently, or until the leaves are wilted. While you broil the sardines, sprinkle with the pine nuts and keep warm.
3. The broiler should be set at high. Aluminum foil should be used to line the broiler pan. Lightly grease the foil. Place the sardines in a line on the pan and 4 inches below the heat. For 112 minutes, broil. To flip the sh, use a spatula. Boil for 112 minutes, until the meat is cooked through and the flesh readily flakes, brushing with oil halfway through.
4. Serve the sardines accompanied by the Mediterranean spinach.

# 34. Fruity Yogurt
Time: 20 minutes

Calories: 98 kcal | Fat: 3 grams |Carbohydrates: 15 grams |Protein: 2 grams

## Ingredients:
- ❖ 470ml of yogurt
- ❖ 20g finely grated orange rind
- ❖ 250g of mixed berries, such as blueberries, raspberries, and strawberries, plus extra to decorate
- ❖ Fresh mint sprigs, to decorate (optional)

## Directions:
1. At least two hours before freezing this dish, set the freezer to rapid freezing. Use 12 paper cupcake liners to line a 12-cup muffin pan or 12 small ramekins set on a baking sheet. In a big bowl, combine the yogurt and orange rind.
2. Slice any extra-large strawberries into pieces the same size as the blueberries and raspberries. Yogurt and fruit should be combined before being spooned into ramekins or paper cups. 2 hours or until barely frozen, freeze.
3. If using, garnish with additional fruit and mint sprigs before serving. Don't forget to place the freezer back to its initial position after finished.

# 35. Spiced Banana Milkshake

Time: 10 minutes

Calories: 722 kcal |fat: 41 grams |Carbohydrates: 73 grams |Protein: 14 grams

**Ingredients:**
- ❖ 350ml of skim milk
- ❖ 2 bananas
- ❖ 150ml of yogurt
- ❖ 2g allspice, and a pinch of allspice, to decorate
- ❖ 6 ice cubes (optional)

**Directions:**
1. Place the milk, bananas, yogurt, and allspice in a blender and process gently until smooth.
2. Pour the mixture into two glasses and serve with ice, if using. Add a pinch of allspice to decorate.

# 36. Chicken and Barley Stew

Time: 55 minutes

Calories: 132 grams |fat: 2.3 grams |Carbohydrates: 21 grams |Protein: 7.3 grams

## Ingredients:

- ❖ 30ml of vegetable oil
- ❖ 8 small, skinless chicken thighs
- ❖ Chicken stock
- ❖ 120g barley, rinsed and drained
- ❖ 6 small new potatoes, unpeeled and halved lengthwise
- ❖ 2 large carrots, sliced
- ❖ 1 leek, sliced
- ❖ 2 shallots, sliced

- ❖ 10g tomato paste
- ❖ 1 bay leaf
- ❖ 1 zucchini, sliced
- ❖ 25g of chopped fresh at-leaf parsley, plus extra sprigs to garnish
- ❖ 10g all-purpose flour
- ❖ 25ml water
- ❖ Salt and pepper

## Directions:

1. In a big casserole dish, heat the oil over medium heat. Add the chicken and cook it for 3 minutes before flipping it over and cooking it for a further 2 minutes on the other side. Add the tomato paste, bay leaf, barley, potatoes, carrots, leeks, and shallots to the dish. Boil for a few minutes, then turn down the heat and simmer for 30 minutes.
2. Include the zucchini and parsley, cover the pan, and simmer it for an additional 20 minutes, or until the chicken is cooked through and the juices flow clear when the tip of a knife is pushed into the thickest portion of the meat. Remove and discard the bay leaf.
3. Combine the flour and water in a another basin and stir to form a smooth paste. It should be added to the stew and cooked for an additional five minutes while stirring. Add salt and pepper to taste.
4. Take the pot off the heat, spoon the soup into serving cups, and top with fresh parsley sprigs.

# 37. Apple and Oat Muffins
Time: 40 minutes

Calories: 159.4 kcal |fat: 3.6 grams |Carbohydrates: 31.1 grams |Protein: 4.3 grams

## Ingredients:
- 125g all-purpose flour
- 12g baking powder
- 2g ground allspice
- 200g firmly packed light brown sugar
- 250g of rolled oats
- 1 large apple unpeeled
- 2 eggs
- 100ml skim milk
- 100ml fresh apple juice
- 100ml sunflower oil

## Directions:
1. Set the oven to 205°C for starters. Use baking cups to line a 12-cup muffin pan. In a big bowl, sift together the flour, baking soda, and allspice. Add the sugar and 112 cups of the oats by stirring.
2. Remove the apple cores and cut the fruit finely. Stir together after adding to the flour mixture.
3. Whisk the milk, apple juice, and oil into the eggs in a bowl after lightly beating them. The beaten liquid ingredients should be added to a well you've created in the middle of the dry ingredients. Don't overmix; gently stir until barely incorporated.
4. Fill the muffin tray with the prepared batter. Over the muffin tops, strew the remaining oats. Bake for about 20 minutes in a preheated oven, or until the bread is well-risen, golden brown, and firm to the touch.
5. Serve the muffins warm or transfer them to a wire rack to cool entirely after cooling in the pan for 5 minutes.

# 38. Brown Rice Salad and Spicy Chickpea

Time: 45 minutes

Calories: 465 kcal |fat: 22.9 grams |Carbohydrates: 61.5 grams |Protein: 8.8 grams

## Ingredients:

- 10ml of olive oil
- 13g of cumin seeds, gently crushed
- 7g of coriander seeds, gently crushed
- 1 red onion, sliced
- 8g of garam masala (you can create your own by combining equal parts of ground cumin, black pepper, cloves, and nutmeg. It is available in Asian grocery stores.)
- 300g of brown rice
- 70g of raisins
- 800ml of simmering vegetable stock
- 425g of can chickpeas, drained and rinsed
- 80g of chopped fresh cilantro, plus extra sprigs to garnish
- 25g of slivered almonds
- 350g of drained and crumbled feta cheese, to serve

## Directions:

1. To the warm olive oil in a saucepan, add the cumin and coriander seeds. Cook the onion for one minute before adding it. After the onion has been cooking for two to three minutes, stir in the garam masala. The spices are completely combined, then the rice and raisins are added.
2. Bring the mixture to a boil after adding the stock. Reduce the heat, cover the pan, and simmer for 25 minutes after the rice is cooked and all the stock has been absorbed.
3. Combine the drained chickpeas, finely chopped cilantro, and almond slivers. To serve warm or cold, take the casserole off the stove, transfer it to serving dishes, top with crumbled feta cheese, and fresh cilantro.

# 39. Kidney Bean Risotto

Time: 1 hour 15 minutes

Calories: 290 kcal |fat: 4.5 grams |Carbohydrates: 52 grams |Protein: 8 grams

## Ingredients:

- 60ml ofolive oil
- 1 onion, chopped
- 2 garlic cloves, nely chopped
- 200g of brown rice
- About 600ml of simmering vegetable stock
- 1 red bell pepper, seeded and chopped
- 2 celery stalks, sliced
- 400g of thinly sliced cremini mushrooms
- 1 can red kidney beans, drained and rinsed
- 40g of chopped fresh parsley, plus extra to garnish
- 60g of cashew nuts
- Salt and pepper

## Directions:

1. In a big, heavy pot, heat half the oil. Add the onion and simmer for 5 minutes, or until softened, stirring regularly. Add the rice and toss for 1 minute, or until the grains are well-coated with oil. Add the remaining half of the garlic and cook, stirring often, for 2 minutes.
2. Stirring constantly, add the stock and a pinch of salt. Bring to a boil. Simmer for 35–40 minutes, covered, or until all the liquid has been absorbed.
3. In the meantime, warm the rest of the oil in a large skillet. Cook the bell pepper and celery for 5 minutes while stirring constantly. Cook, stirring constantly for 4-5 minutes, the remaining garlic and the cut mushrooms.
4. Add the rice to the skillet and stir. Beans, parsley, and cashews should all be added. Add salt and pepper, then cook while stirring constantly until heated. Place in a serving dish, cover with more parsley, and serve right away.

# 40. Lemon Balm Loaf

Time: 1 hour 10 minutes

Calories: 229 kcal |fat: 9 grams |Carbohydrates: 35 grams |Protein: 3 grams

## Ingredients:
- ❖ Butter, for greasing
- ❖ 330g of whole-wheat flour
- ❖ 7g of baking powder
- ❖ 109g of sugar
- ❖ Grated rind of half a lemon
- ❖ 25g of chopped lemon balm leaves
- ❖ 150ml of plain yogurt
- ❖ 150ml of peanut oil
- ❖ 3 eggs, beaten
- ❖ 150ml of blueberries

## Directions:
1. Set the oven to 190°C for starters. An 812-inch loaf pan should be greased and lined with parchment paper.
2. Combine the dry ingredients, lemon rind, and chopped lemon balm in a sizable basin.
3. Beat the eggs, oil, and plain yogurt together before combining them with the dry ingredients.
4. After gently bursting the blueberries, add them into the cake batter.
5. After mixing the batter, pour it into the pan that has been prepared. Bake for an hour, or until a fork inserted in the center comes out clean. Before serving, take out of the pan and let cool on a wire rack.

# 41. Mushroom and Rosemary Stroganoff
Time: 20 minutes

Calories: 193 kcal | fat: 11.25 grams |Carbohydrates: 16.25 grams |Protein: 6.75 grams

## Ingredients:
- ❖ 30ml of olive oil
- ❖ 1 large onion, diced
- ❖ 2 garlic doves, nely chopped
- ❖ 1 leek, diced
- ❖ 1 pound wild mushrooms, coarsely chopped
- ❖ 3 large portobello mushrooms, sliced
- ❖ 25g of paprika
- ❖ 25g of chopped fresh rosemary
- ❖ Juice from half a lemon
- ❖ 120ml of simmering vegetable stock
- ❖ 25g of crème fraîche or sour cream
- ❖ Salt and pepper
- ❖ Cooked brown rice, to serve

## Directions:
1. In a sizable saucepan with hot oil, soften the onion, garlic, and leek.
2. Mix well after adding the mushrooms and paprika.
3. Cook for a few minutes after adding the rosemary and lemon juice.
4. Add the vegetable stock, then boil the mixture until the liquid has been cut in half.
5. Add the crème fraîche and season with salt and pepper before serving with just-made rice.

# 42. Sage Risotto

Time: 50 minutes

Calories: 150 kcal | fat: 1.5 grams |Carbohydrates: 31 grams |Protein: 4 grams

## Ingredients:
- ❖ About 50g of butter
- ❖ 1 onion, diced
- ❖ 340g of brown rice
- ❖ 40ml of white wine
- ❖ 1.3 liters of simmering vegetable stock
- ❖ 185g of quinoa
- ❖ 10−12 chopped fresh sage leaves
- ❖ 100g of grated Parmesan cheese

## Directions:
1. In a skillet, melt 3 spoons of the butter, then sauté the onion for 5 to 6 minutes, or until tender.
2. After adding the brown rice and cooking it for one to two minutes, add the wine. Pour in the stock and bring to a boil once more when the wine has reduced by half. For 15 minutes, simmer on a lower heat.
3. Stir in the quinoa and sage and cook for another 10−12 minutes, until the liquid has been absorbed and the rice and quinoa are both cooked.
4. Stir in the remaining butter and grated Parmesan cheese. Transfer to serving plates and serve immediately.

# 43. Mushroom with Parsley and Olive Oil
## Time: 20 minutes

Calories: 67 kcal |fat: 6 grams |Carbohydrates: 4 grams |Protein: 3 grams

## Ingredients:

- ❖ 450g of mushrooms
- ❖ 120ml of extra virgin olive oil
- ❖ 2 garlic cloves, neatly chopped
- ❖ Large handful of parsley chopped
- ❖ Salt and pepper
- ❖ Sourdough toast, to serve

## Directions:

1. Distinguish the mushroom stems from the crowns. The stems should be roughly chopped and stored. Add the oil to a skillet and heat it up. Add the mushroom caps and sauté when it's hot. Check the undersides and flip them over if they start to brown. Add salt and pepper to taste.
2. For 5 to 10 minutes, or until the flavors really start to come together and the garlic's bite begins to soften, add the garlic, chopped mushroom stems, and parsley.
3. With a little of the hot oil from the skillet drizzled over them, serve the mushrooms on pieces of sourdough toast.

# 44. Poached Pears in Green Tea

Time: 20 minutes

Calories: 293.6 kcal |fat: 12.9 grams |Carbohydrates: 48.2 grams |Protein: 1.3 grams

## Ingredients:
- 2 slightly underripe pears, halved and peeled
- 10ml of lemon juice
- 800ml of water
- 4 slices of fresh ginger
- 2 star anise
- 1 cinnamon stick
- 10ml of honey
- 2 green tea bags

## Directions:
1. Scoop out the center of each pear using a melon baller or teaspoon. To keep the pears from turning brown, squeeze the lemon juice over them.
2. In a big sauté pan, bring the water to a boil. The ginger, star anise, cinnamon, and honey are added after the heat is reduced to a simmer. Pears are then added after stirring until the honey melts.
3. Use a slotted spoon to remove the pears from the pan after simmering them for 15 to 20 minutes, partially covered, until they are soft. Green tea is added, the heat is slightly raised, and the mixture simmers for about 5 minutes, or until the liquid has decreased and thickened into syrup.
4. Spices and tea bags should be taken out of the cooking syrup. Per person, place 2 pear halves on a plate and cover with syrup.

# 45. Honey and Yogurt Dressing

Time: 10 minutes

Calories: 23 kcal |fat: 0.8 grams |Carbohydrates: 3 grams |Protein: 0.5 grams

## Ingredients:

- ❖ 10ml of honey
- ❖ 80ml of low-fat plain yogurt
- ❖ Pepper and Salt

## Directions:

1. Yogurt and honey should be blended completely with a fork after being placed in a glass bowl. Add salt and pepper to taste.

# 46.Oatmeal with Banana and Pollen

Time: 20 minutes

Calories: 95 kcal |fat: 3 grams |Carbohydrates: 27 grams |Protein: 5 grams

## Ingredients:
- ❖ 300g of rolled oats
- ❖ 700ml of milk
- ❖ 700ml of water
- ❖ 60ml of plain yogurt
- ❖ 3 bananas, sliced
- ❖ 30g of bee pollen grains

## Directions:
1. In a saucepan, combine the oats with the milk and water. Bring to a boil while stirring occasionally.
2. Stirring occasionally, simmer the oatmeal for 8 to 10 minutes or until it thickens. Observe for one minute.
3. Divide the oats among the four dishes for serving. Slices of banana, bee pollen, and a dollop of plain yogurt should be sprinkled on top of each serving of oatmeal.

# 47. Paper Wrapped Rice with nuts

Time: 40 minutes

Calories: 235 kcal |fat: 0.9 grams |Carbohydrates: 50 grams |Protein: 3.8 grams

## Ingredients:

- ❖ 40g of blanched almonds
- ❖ About 30g of pistachio nuts
- ❖ 30ml of honey
- ❖ 300g of fresh bread crumbs
- ❖ Freshly squeezed orange
- ❖ 30ml of sesame oil
- ❖ 4 sheets of paper for wrapping

## Directions:

1. Toast the nuts over medium-high heat in a dry nonstick skillet. Remove from the skillet as soon as they begin to brown.
2. Heat the honey in a saucepan over low heat; add the nuts, bread crumbs, orange zest, and sesame oil. Stir continually for 5 minutes, until the mix thickens to a paste. Remove from the heat and let cool.
3. The rice papers should be spread out on a surface and brushed with warm water; after a few minutes, they will soften and become malleable. Distribute the nut mixture among the rice papers, positioning it in the center in the form of a cylinder. Serve with orange peel garnish after carefully folding the ends over and rolling them up.

# 48. Oat-Nut Mix

Time: 20 minutes

Calories: 110 kcal |fat: 2 grams |Carbohydrates: 19 grams |Protein: 4 grams

## Ingredients:
- ❖ Peanut oil, for brushing
- ❖ About 130g of rolled oats
- ❖ 38g of pine nuts
- ❖ 30g of hazelnuts
- ❖ 30g of almonds
- ❖ 30g of nuts, coarsely chopped
- ❖ 26g of sun seeds
- ❖ 26g of pumpkin seeds
- ❖ 12g of axseeds
- ❖ 40g of chopped dried apricots
- ❖ 40g of golden raisins
- ❖ 12g of cinnamon, ground fine

## Directions:
1. Brush a little oil into a nonstick skillet and heat it up over medium heat. Oats and pine nuts should smell nutty and appear to be beginning to turn golden after 8 to 10 minutes of constant stirring. Cool down.
2. Place the toasted oat mixture in a large bowl and combine with the other ingredients. Keep in an airtight jar in the refrigerator.

# 49. Zucchini-Hazelnut Salad with Cheese Topping

Time: 45 minutes

Calories: 246 kcal |fat: 19 grams |Carbohydrates: 10.1 grams |Protein: 9.3 grams

## Ingredients:

- ❖ 4–6 small zucchini, sliced into thin ribbons
- ❖ Freshly squeezed lemon juice
- ❖ 40ml of olive oil
- ❖ Roughly chopped basil leaves of about 5-8
- ❖ 72g of hazelnuts
- ❖ About 300gof crumbled goat cheese

## Directions:

1. Place the zucchini in a bowl and toss with the lemon juice, olive oil, and basil leaves.
2. Distribute over four plates for serving, then top with goat cheese crumbles and chopped hazelnuts.

# 50. Pecan-Rice Mushrooms

Time: 1 hour 15 minutes

Calories: 160 kcal |fat: 5 grams |Carbohydrates: 35 grams |Protein: 4 grams

## Ingredients:

- ❖ 15ml of olive oil
- ❖ 4 scallions, sliced
- ❖ About 6g of crushed, dried red pepper
- ❖ 4 large portobello mushrooms
- ❖ 100g of long-grain rice

- ❖ About 700ml of simmering vegetable stock
- ❖ 50g of chopped pecans
- ❖ 90g of grated Manchego cheese
- ❖ 13 g chopped fresh parsley

## Directions:

1. Preheat the oven to 175°C.
2. Scallions and red pepper flakes should be cooked in hot oil for one to two minutes.
3. Cut off the mushroom stems before chopping and adding them to the onion mixture. Cook for two minutes. Before adding vegetable stock and putting to a boil, the rice needs to be thoroughly mixed together. Reduce the heat after the rice has finished cooking, then simmer it for 25 minutes.
4. The mushroom caps should be placed on a baking sheet and baked for 10 minutes in a preheated oven.
5. Cooked rice is mixed with pecans, Manchego cheese, parsley, and spice before being spooned over the mushrooms and piled on top of each one. After 10 minutes of baking, serve right away.

# 51. Sauteed Spinach and Kale

Time: 30 mins

Serving size: 4 | Calories: 118 | Fat: 9g | Carbohydrates: 8g | Protein: 3g

**Ingredients:**
- 15ml of Extra Virgin Olive Oil
- 1/2 of a medium onion
- 1 minced garlic clove
- 120g of spinach
- 120g of  Kale
- 115g of lemon juice
- 82g of sweet corn
- 30g of roasted pine nuts
- pepper and salt to taste

**Directions:**
1. In a sauté pan, heat the olive oil over medium-high heat for about a minute.
2. Add the onions and stir. When the onions are transparent, add the minced garlic. After another minute, then you'll start adding the spinach and kale in small batches, making sure to stir the greens between additions. Add more when the vegetables wilt and simmer down. Then add the remaining kale and spinach after that. Cook for approximately 7 minutes, or until all of the leaves have softened.
3. When you're satisfied with the softness of the greens, remove your pan from heat. Then add lemon juice, and stir it in.
4. To taste, mix in salt and pepper. Add sweet corn and pine nuts on top and serve.

# 52. Green Shakshuka

Time: 40 mins

Serving: 3 | Calories: 355 | Fat: 30g | Carbohydrates: 19g | Protein: 19g

## Ingredients:

- ❖ 10ml of olive oil
- ❖ 1 big onion, chopped
- ❖ 4 garlic cloves, minced
- ❖ 1 medium zucchini, diced
- ❖ 2g Cumin
- ❖ 2g of coriander
- ❖ 3g sea salt
- ❖ 0.5g ground pepper
- ❖ 120g baby spinach
- ❖ 120g cups kale,
- ❖ 1/2 lemon juice
- ❖ 4-5 eggs
- ❖ 8g finely chopped cilantro
- ❖ 60g feta cheese,
- ❖ 1 Medium sized avocado
- ❖ 1 green onions, diced

## Directions:

1. First, we must heat up our olive oil. Set the stove to medium heat. A big skillet is used to heat the oil for about two minutes.
2. Add the chopped onion to the heated oil and Cook the onion in the skillet for 5 to 10 minutes, or until it is tender and fragrant. Sauté for an additional 2–3 minutes after adding the zucchini and garlic.
3. Add Salt, pepper, coriander, and cumin. After giving the mixture a swirl, heat it for an additional minute. Kale and spinach are chopped and added to the mixture in the skillet a cup at a time, stirring continuously until the spinach and kale start to wilt/soften. After this, Stir in the lemon juice.
2. Create 4-5 holes in the greens mixture and turn the heat down to low. Crack an egg into each well and cover the pan. Cook for approval five minutes or until the egg whites are fully cooked.
6. Turn off the heat, uncover the skillet, sprinkle the feta cheese and cilantro on top, and let everything settle for a couple of minutes before serving.
7. Place a large quantity of greens and 1-2 eggs on each plate. Add more feta cheese, fresh cilantro, green onions, and avocado as garnishes. For a complete meal, serve with toast, vegetables, or over a nutritious grain like quinoa or brown rice.

# 53. Creamed Lacinato Kale

Time: 45 mins

Serving: 6 | Calories: 400 | Fat: 35g | Carbohydrates: 20 | Protein: 25g

## Ingredients:

- 30ml of Extra virgin olive oil,
- 450g of finely chopped fresh lacinato
- 280g of dry frozen spinach.
- 480g of heavy cream
- 30g of finely shredded Parmesan
- 15g of Grated Gruyere
- 51g Worcestershire sauce
- 0.5g Red chile flakes
- 0.5g teaspoon of ground nutmeg
- 1 small sized lemon
- 30g panko breadcrumbs
- Salt to taste

## Directions:

1. Set the oven to 177 degrees Celsius
2. In a big pan, heat 1 tablespoon of oil over high heat. Add half of the kale to the pan once the oil starts to smoke. Add salt, stir, and simmer for 2 to 3 minutes, or until the leaves become a deep green color and lose 50% to 75% of their volume. Then add more oil, spinach and kale to the pan. Repeat the process, adding more greens and oil to the bowl as you go.
3. Add the cream and the increase oven to a high heat. Simmer the mixture For about 5 minutes, simmer the cream until it has reduced in mass.
2. Add the salt to taste along with the Parmesan, Gruyere, Worcestershire, chili flakes, nutmeg, and lemon zest and juice.
8. Add the cooked greens onto a baking pan, sprinkle the panko on top and bake for 12 to 15 minutes, or until heated.
9. Serve as desired.

# 54. Green Smoothie

Time: 10 mins

Serving: 4 | Calories: 64 | Fat: 20g | Carbohydrates: 13g | Protein: 2g

## Ingredients:

- ❖ 1 serving baby spinach
- ❖ 30g of kale with the stems removed
- ❖ 3/4 medium sized pineapple
- ❖ 1 green apple
- ❖ 1 very large, ripe banana
- ❖ 1/2 ginger (peeled)
- ❖ 15ml Lemon juice
- ❖ Oat milk, or coconut milk.
- ❖ several ice cubes
- ❖ 3g of parsley leaves

## Directions:

1. Fill your blender jar with a large amount of kale and spinach. Include the green apple and pineapple. Add a ripe banana that has been peeled. Add parsley leaves and peeled ginger.
2. Then add your lemon juice, oat milk or coconut milk. The amount you'll add will depend on your desired consistency. Add ice.
3. Thoroughly blend all the components for at least two minutes. Then pour your smoothie into a container.
4. Sprinkle Chia seeds on top of the green smoothie and serve chilled.

# 55. Green Smoothie with Grapefruit

Time: 10 mins

Serving: 2 | Calories: 60 | Fat: 15g | Carbohydrates: 14g | Protein: 5g

**Ingredients:**
- ❖ 30g spinach
- ❖ 1/2 large banana
- ❖ 60g Unsweetened oat milk
- ❖ 1g teaspoon ginger, grated
- ❖ 10g of hemp seeds
- ❖ 5g protein powder
- ❖ 1/3 of a medium grapefruit
- ❖ 1 large green apple

**Directions:**
1. Fill up your blender jar with a large amount of kale. Include the green apple and grapefruit. Add your peeled banana and ginger.
2. Scoop Ina your protein powder and unsweetened oat milk.
3. Thoroughly blend all the components for at least two minutes. Then pour your smoothie into a container and serve.

# 56. Quinoa Salad

Time: 30 mins

Serving: 4 | Calories: 300 | Fat: 19g | Carbohydrates: 27g | Protein: 17g

## Ingredients:

- 185g Quinoa
- 8g cup Coriander leaves
- 3 garlic cloves, minced
- 30ml of olive oil

- 15ml of lemon juice
- 15ml Vinegar
- 3g Salt
- 230g of water

## For the quinoa Salad:

- 10g coriander leaves
- 30g finely sliced carrots
- 20g chopped red and green bell peppers

- 1 cucumber, chopped
- 60g chopped roasted peanuts.

## Directions:

1. Rinse the Quinoa twice and drain. Place the drained quinoa in a pan with the water, salt, and bring to a boil. Cook with the lid on for 15 minutes, or until the water is absorbed. The cooked quinoa will have a fluffy appearance.
2. In a different bowl, Combine cilantro, olive oil, lemon juice, and vinegar in a bowl. This is the dressing. Put that aside.
3. To your cooked quinoa, add carrot, bell pepper, onion, cucumber, peanuts, cilantro and the dressing.
4. Mix together. You can either serve it right now or store it in the fridge until you're ready to do so.

# 57. Quinoa salad with Honey Lemon Mint vinaigrette

Time: 20 mins

Serving: 8 | Calories: 800 | Fat: 30g | Carbohydrates: 120g | Protein: 27g

## Ingredients:

- 550g cooked quinoa
- 30g thinly sliced scallions
- 60g of dried cranberries
- 1 large Granny Smith apple, chopped
- 30g cup roasted almonds, chopped

## For the honey lemon mint vinaigrette:

- 60g Lemon juice
- 6g of hot water
- 4g of fresh mint
- 45ml of honey
- 54g of Extra virgin olive oil
- Kosher salt
- Ground black pepper

## Directions:

1. Combine the honey, lemon juice, olive oil, mint, and warm water in a small mixing bowl or blender. Use salt and pepper to season the vinaigrette mixture.
2. Apples, roasted almonds, scallions, and dried cranberries should all be added to cooked quinoa in a different pan.
3. Before serving, sprinkle the quinoa salad with 1/2 cup of the prepared vinaigrette and mix well.

# 58. Quinoa Cauliflower Chowder
Time: 1 hour

Serving: 6 | Calories: 600 | Fat: 26g | Carbohydrates: 80g | Protein: 27g

## Ingredients:
- 90g coarsely chopped cauliflower
- 10g of butter
- 185g Quinoa
- 2 garlic cloves, minced
- 1 red bell pepper, chopped
- 1 carrot, diced
- 1 peeled and diced potato
- 440ml vegetable broth
- 470ml of milk
- 15g kosher salt
- 4g dried thyme,
- 4g dried bay leaves

## Directions:
1. Melt 2 tablespoons of butter in a big Dutch oven over medium-high heat. Add and Cook the garlic until it becomes fragrant. Add the carrots and red bell pepper and cook for 10 minutes.
2. Add the potato, cauliflower, milk, bay leaf, thyme, and kosher salt along with the vegetable broth. Bring to a boil, then lower the heat to a simmer for about 10 to 12 minutes on low heat.
5. Rinse the quinoa in cold water, then put it in a small pan and add 2 cups of cold water to cover. Add kosher salt to taste and bring to a boil. Cook the quinoa until tender after reducing the heat to a simmer. With a fork, fluff and reserve.
6. Into a high-power blender, add 3 cups of vegetable broth and vegetables, primarily potatoes and cauliflower, and blend till smooth. Some vegetables should remain in the pot for texture.
7. Remove the bay leaves from the simmering mixture, then add the blended mixture into it. Cook for 5 minutes
8. Add the remaining butter and the cooked quinoa. Quinoa absorbs some moisture, which causes it to thicken soup when combined with butter. Serve right away.

# 59. Caribbean Salmon Quinoa bowl

Time: 30 mins

Serving: 4 | Calories: 439 | Fat: 13g | Carbohydrates: 54g | Protein: 28g

## Ingredients:

- 370g cooked quinoa
- 120g of rinsed and drained canned black beans

- For salmon Fillet
- 4 fillets of wild salmon
- 6g chili powder

- 0.5g of cinnamon powder
- 0.5g coriander powder
- 0.5g cayenne
- 2g cumin, ground
- 1g of an allspice berry
- Ground black pepper
- Pinch of salt.

## For the Salsa Mango:

- 2 medium sized mangos, diced
- 10g cup minced cilantro
- 20g cup red onion
- 2ml lime, juiced

- 0.5g chili powder
- Salt

## Directions:

1. All the salmon fillet seasonings should be combined in a small basin. Rub the salmon with a uniform distribution of the spice mixture.
2. Put the fillets on a grill that has been greased and heated to a medium-high temperature. Cook the salmon on the grill for 4 to 6 minutes, or until it flakes when examined with a fork.
3. Thoroughly mix all of the ingredients for the mango salsa in a medium bowl until well blended.
4. Place 1 salmon fillet, black beans, cooked quinoa, and a portion of the mango salsa in 4 dishes and serve.

# 60. Grilled Salmon with Mango Cucumber Mint Salsa

Time: 25 mins

Serving: 4 | Calories: 302 | Fat: 14g | Carbohydrates: 24g | Protein: 19g

## Ingredients:

- 1/2 medium sized cucumber, with the seeds removed and diced
- 18g red onion, chopped
- 1 minced, seeded, and stemmed jalapeno
- 6ml lime juice,
- 20g olive oil
- 2 teaspoons of freshly chopped mint
- 4 salmon fillets
- Ground black pepper to taste
- salt to taste
- 2 mangos, peeled and diced

## Directions:

1. Heat the grill to a medium-high setting and grease the grill grates with a brush. Spice your salmon with salt and pepper and grill for 3–4 minutes, flipping it once or until the internal temperature reaches 50 degrees Celsius
2. Add all of the salsa's ingredients to a medium bowl. I added about a 1/2 teaspoon of kosher salt and stirred everything together and your grilled fish.
3. Serve.

# 61. Greek Salmon Salad with Tahini Yogurt Dressing

Time: 2.5 hours

Serving: 4 | Calories: 361 | Fat: 21g | Carbohydrates: 11g | Protein: 33g

## Ingredients:

### For the Salmon:
- 4 (113g each) skin-on wild salmon fillets
- 2g each of dill and oregano
- 2g of garlic granules
- To taste, add freshly ground black pepper and kosher salt.

### For the Tahini Yogurt Dressing:
- 120g unsweetened Greek yogurt
- 25ml of olive oil
- 6g tahini
- One lemon, juiced
- 2g cumin powder
- 2g grated garlic
- 2g dried dill
- 2g Coriander
- To taste, add freshly ground black pepper and kosher salt.

### For the Salad:
- 180g of romaine lettuce, chopped
- 40g of red onion, thinly sliced
- 40g Kalamata olives
- 1 big cucumber, sliced
- 57g of cubed feta cheese
- 60g of cherry tomatoes
- 20g of olive oil
- 2ml Red wine vinegar
- 0.5g Oregano, dry
- 0.5g dried dill
- To taste, add black pepper and kosher salt.

## Directions:

1. Use the olive oil to grease the grill grates and heat them to a medium-high temperature. While the grill is heating up, add all the salmon's spices into a mortar and use the pestle or your hands to grind/mix them.
2. Sprinkle the mixed spices on the Salmon fillet. Grill the salmon fillet for 3 to 5 minutes per side, although this time is dependent on the thickness of your fish. The thicker the fish, the more time it'll take to grill. Remove the grilled salmon off the grill, let them sit for a while, before skinning them then using a fork to pieces it.
4. For the Tahini Yogurt Dressing, gather all of the dressing's components in a small bowl and stir until well mixed. Add enough salt and pepper till you're satisfied with the taste. Next, keep it in the fridge until when you want to serve.

5. Then, Mix all the salad ingredients except the romaine lettuce. Mix them by tossing, till all the ingredients are thoroughly mixed.
6. The romaine lettuce should be added to a dish. Also add the salmon, olives, feta, and cucumber mixture to the lettuce. Add the dressing on top and serve.

## 62. Quinoa Vegetable Soup with Kale

Time: 3 hours

Serving: 4 | Calories: 280 | Fat: 10.3g | Carbohydrates: 10.3g | Protein: 9g

**Ingredients:**

- ❖ 15ml Extra virgin olive oil
- ❖ 60g chopped seasonal vegetables, such as zucchini, yellow squash, bell pepper, sweet potatoes, or butternut squash;
- ❖ 1 medium white onion
- ❖ 3 carrots
- ❖ 2 celery stalks;
- ❖ 6 garlic cloves, minced
- ❖ 1g dried thyme
- ❖ 1 large can diced tomatoes
- ❖ 920ml vegetable broth
- ❖ 460g of water
- ❖ 6g salt; add more if you want
- ❖ 1 bay leaf,
- ❖ Red pepper flakes with a pinch
- ❖ black pepper freshly ground
- ❖ 1 can washed and drained chickpeas
- ❖ 30g freshly cut collard greens.
- ❖ 185g of quinoa
- ❖ 6ml lemon juice to taste
- ❖ Finely grated Parmesan cheese to garnish.

**Directions:**

1. Rinse 1 cup of quinoa thoroughly in a colander with fine mesh (use less for a lighter, more broth-y soup)
2. Over medium heat, warm the olive oil in a sizable Dutch oven. Seasonal vegetables, diced onion, carrot, and celery, as well as a bit of salt, are added while the oil is shimmering. Cook while frequently stirring for about 6 to 8 minutes, or until the onion has softened and is beginning to turn translucent.
3. Add the thyme and garlic. Cook for approximately a minute, stirring regularly, until aromatic. Add the diced tomatoes and their liquids, stirring often for a few more minutes.
4. Add the water, broth, and quinoa. Add two bay leaves, one teaspoon of salt, and a dash of red pepper flakes. Add a lot of freshly ground black pepper to the dish.

Increase the heat to bring the mixture to a boil, then lower the heat, partially cover the pot, and keep a slow simmer.

5.  Remove the lid and add the beans and the chopped greens after 25 minutes of cooking. Keep the greens boiling for another five minutes or so, or until they are soft enough for you.

6.  After turning off the heat, take the bay leaves out of the saucepan. Add 1 tsp. of lemon juice and stir. Taste and season with extra salt, pepper, and/or lemon juice until the flavors actually come together. Garnish with freshly grated Parmesan.

# 63. Scrumptious quinoa and zucchini loaf

Time: 1 hour 15 mins

Serving: 4 | Calories: 234 | Fat: 7.2g | Carbohydrates: 36.7g | Protein: 9g

## Ingredients:

- 8g of toasted sesame seeds
- 120g of rolled oats
- 10g thyme
- 30g of Sumac
- 2g Baking powder
- 12g sea salt

- 6g Psyllium husk
- 50 g of almond meal
- 370g cooked quinoa
- 2 grated zucchinis
- 3 lightly whisked eggs

## Directions:

1. Oven: Preheat to 190 C
2. Add Oats, sesame seeds, and thyme to a food processor or blender and pulsed a few times to break them up.
3. Transferring them to a bowl, mix them thoroughly with the remaining dry ingredients. Squeeze as much juice as you can out of the zucchini, and then combine it with the quinoa in the dry mixture. After combining, gently mix in the whisked eggs.
4. Place the mixture in a lined loaf pan, and if preferred, garnish with sesame seeds or rolled oats.
5. Bake for 35 to 40 minutes, or until thoroughly done. Allow it cool in the tin before transferring to a cooling rack.

# 64. Lemon, Olive, and Parsley Quinoa Cakes
Time: 1 hour 30 mins

Serving: 4 | Calories: 200 | Fat: 8.3g | Carbohydrates: 22.4g | Protein: 9.6g

## Ingredients:
- 520g uncooked quinoa
- 60ml water
- 3g salt
- 4 big eggs, beaten
- 1 medium yellow onion, chopped
- 4 garlic cloves, chopped
- 1/2 grated parmesan cheese
- 1/3 olives, chopped
- 1/3 chopped parsley
- 2g of lemon zest
- 59g of breadcrumbs
- 3g of salt
- 1g coarsely powdered black pepper
- 30ml of olive oil
- 10ml of water

## Directions:
1. Place dry quinoa in a fine-mesh strainer and give it a few minutes to soak in lukewarm water.
2. In a medium saucepan, combine the quinoa, water, and 1/2 teaspoon salt. On medium heat, stir and gently boil for about 25 to 30 minutes, or until the quinoa is soft. Let it simmer, covered over low heat. After removing from the heat, let the food cool to room temperature.
3. Whisk eggs in a small bowl. Place aside.
4. Combine the cooled quinoa with the onion, garlic, cheese, olives, parsley, lemon zest, and seasonings in a sizable bowl. Once the quinoa is evenly seasoned, whisk in the eggs. To completely moisten the mixture, add water. To prevent quinoa from drying out when cooking, it should be slightly moist.
6. Scoop out the mixture in 2 tablespoon portions. Make a patty by shaping with clean, moist fingertips.
7. Heat olive oil in a big skillet over a medium heat. Drop patties directly into the heated skillet. Fill the heating skillet with four to six patties (or as many as you can fit without overloading). To correctly turn them, you'll need a little space.
8. Cook for 4 to 5 minutes on each side, or until each side is wonderfully browned. Internal cooking is facilitated by medium-low heat. Repeat with the remaining quinoa mixture after removing the browned cakes to a plate lined with paper towels. Serve hot.

# 65. Five Minutes Parfait

Time: 5 mins

Serving: 4 | Calories: 260 | Fat: 2.8g | Carbohydrates: 49.8g | Protein: 9.8g

## Ingredients:

- ❖ 140g Greek yogurt, plain
- ❖ 80g of cooked quinoa
- ❖ 9g of honey
- ❖ 40g Cheerios + Ancient Grains cereal
- ❖ 60g pomegranate seeds

## Directions:

1. Add the quinoa, honey, and Greek yogurt, in that order.
2. In the base of a circular glass, distribute half of the yogurt mixture. Repeat layering once more, covering with half of the cereal and half of the pomegranate arils. Serve right away.

# 66. Chicken Quinoa Chilli

Time: 10 hours

Serving: 6 | Calories: 364 | Fat: 6.4g | Carbohydrates: 59.9g | Protein: 23.4g

## Ingredients:

- 790g can diced tomatoes
- 395g diced tomatoes with green chilies,
- 425g each of rinsed and drained black beans, corn and chili beans
- 460g of chicken stock
- 3 little boneless, skinless chicken breasts
- 12g Garlic powder
- 6g of powdered onion
- 4g Cumin
- 1g Red pepper flakes
- 6g Chili powder
- 185g of rinsed quinoa
- Topping of your choice (cheese, sour cream, avocados, and tortilla strips)

## Directions:

1. Before adding everything to a 6-quart slow cooker, make sure the quinoa has been thoroughly rinsed. Then add your chicken.

2. Cook for 4-6 hours on high or 6-8 hours on low. You might need to cook the chicken for longer if it's frozen.

3. With two forks, remove the chicken and shred it. Add cheese, sour cream, avocados, and tortilla strips as a garnish.

# 67. Quinoa-based Cream of Mushroom Soup

Time: 2 hours 30 mins

Serving: 5 | Calories: 409 | Fat: 12.5g | Carbohydrates: 59.9g | Protein: 15.7g

## Ingredients:

- 370g cooked quinoa white
- 90g of uncooked cashews
- 2 fresh cremini and a handful of dried shiitake mushrooms
- 920g of vegetable broth
- 2g Oregano, dry
- 6g of dried thyme
- 1 white onion
- 3 celery stalks
- 1 big carrot
- Pepper and salt to taste
- 50 ml of white wine
- 45ml of soy sauce
- 12g of flour (optional)
- shallots for a garnish

## Directions:

1. In a covered pan, combine 2 parts water with 1 part rinsed quinoa to cook the grain. Simmer the mixture until the water is completely absorbed.
2. Additionally, start soaking the raw cashews in warm water to soften them before blending them into a cream later on.
4. Add the mushroom slices, vegetable broth, oregano, and thyme to a stockpot and heat to a simmer. As a result, the soup will be considerably more flavorful and the flavor of the mushrooms will be infused into the broth.
5. Add two cup of fresh cremini and a handful of dried shiitake. Use roughly a third less dry mushrooms because they will expand.
3. The carrots, celery, and onions should be finely diced before being added to a bigger stockpot with a little water. Until the vegetables are tender and the onions are transparent, sauté over medium heat. After that, add 1/2 cup of white wine and boil everything for an additional 5 minutes.
4. After draining the cashews of their soaking liquid, mix them until fully smooth with 1 cup of new water. Then add broth, mushrooms, quinoa, and cashew cream to the large stockpot with the vegetables. Add 3 tablespoons of soy sauce as well.
5. Add 2 teaspoons of flour to the soup and whisk it in rapidly to avoid clumps if you prefer your soup to be thicker. If not, simply simmer it for another 15 minutes or so until it is the ideal consistency.
6. Serve with finely chopped chives.

# 68. General Tso's Tofu and Broccoli

Time: 1 hour

Serving: 4 | Calories: 300 | Fat: 21 g | Carbohydrates: 19 g | Protein: 22g

## Ingredients:

- 450g Firm Tofu
- 60g of cornmeal
- 12g whole grain flour
- 2g of salt
- 1g Black pepper,
- 1g of garlic powder
- 120g soy sauce
- 10ml of rice wine vinegar
- 30ml maple syrup
- 2g of flakes of red pepper
- 1g of smoked paprika
- 2 minced garlic cloves
- 3 onions green
- 2 cups broccoli
- 6g sesame seeds
- 360g brown rice

## Directions:

1. Cut the tofu into tiny chicken-like pieces. Then, combine the cornmeal, flour, salt, black pepper, and garlic powder to produce a mixture. Place each piece of tofu in your air fryer after dipping it in the batter (it should still be moist) or a baking sheet in the oven. Cook the coated pieces at roughly 190 °C until the batter is extremely crispy and brown.
2. Combine in a small bowl soy sauce, rice wine vinegar, and maple syrup in equal amounts, along with some minced garlic, red pepper flakes, and smoky paprika.
3. Sauté the finished dish once the tofu is crispy. Add all the sauce, some frozen and microwaved broccoli florets (preferably previously cooked), chopped green onions, and the tofu nuggets to a big pan. Repeatedly toss until evenly coated, then boil for 5-7 minutes over medium heat.
4. Serve with brown rice and a sprinkle of sesame seeds as a garnish. Any leftovers should be kept in the refrigerator for a minimum of two days.

# 69. Garlic Butter Shrimp Quinoa

Time: 50 mins

Serving: 8 | Calories: 298 | Fat: 13.5g | Carbohydrates: 62g | Protein: 15.8g

## Ingredients:

- 15ml of olive oil
- 1/2 onion, chopped finely
- 5 garlic cloves, minced
- 370g of raw quinoa
- 2g of chili powder
- 920ml chicken or veggie broth
- 90g of salted butter
- 450g Raw shrimp
- pepper and salt as desired
- fresh parsley and lemon juice for serving

## Directions:

1. In a sizable nonstick pot, heat the oil over medium-high heat. Add the onion and cook for about 5 minutes, or until tender. To prevent burning, add 2 teaspoons of the garlic and sauté for 1 minute while stirring continuously.
2. Add 1/2 teaspoon of chili powder along with the uncooked quinoa. Add salt and pepper to taste. To flavor the quinoa, sauté for one additional minute. Add the broth, raise the temperature to a boil, cover, and simmer for 15 to 20 minutes. The quinoa will be completely soft when it is finished. Toss with freshly minced parsley after fluffing with a fork.
3. 1 tablespoon of butter should be melted over medium-high heat in a big skillet while the quinoa is cooking. Add the shrimp and the remaining 1/2 teaspoon chili powder to the skillet with the shrimp once it is heated and the butter has melted. Add salt and pepper, then cook until the outside is golden brown and the inside is no longer translucent. Add 1 teaspoon of garlic and stir it about in the pan until it is very aromatic right before the sauté comes to a close.
5. To make a sauce for drizzling, melt the remaining 5 tablespoons of butter with the 2 teaspoons of garlic paste.
6. Serve the quinoa and shrimp in the same dish, and if wanted, garnish with freshly cut parsley and lemon juice. Pour the melted and slightly cooled butter over the quinoa and shrimp. Serve when still.

# 70. Avocado & Quinoa Stuffed Acorn Squash

Time: 1 hour 30mins

Serving: 8 | Calories: 575 | Fat: 20.8g | Carbohydrates: 70g | Protein: 21.1g

## Ingredients:

- 4 tiny acorn squash, halved
- 30ml Olive oil, extra virgin,
- 1 small onion
- 3 garlic cloves
- 10g cup cumin
- 2g of cilantro
- 1 can of green chilies
- 340g cooked quinoa
- 400g can rinsed and drained black beans
- 30g cup of scallions, chopped
- 30g cup lightly toast pepitas
- 4 feta cheese cubes (optional)
- 2 diced avocados
- 5ml Lemon juice
- freshly ground black pepper and sea salt

## Directions:

1. Set oven to 205 degrees Celsius.
2. Scoop out the insides of an acorn squash by cutting it in half. Add salt and pepper and drizzle with olive oil. Roast the squash cut side up for 35 to 50 minutes, or until it is cooked through and browned on the sides.
3. In the interim, warm the oil in a big skillet over medium heat. Add a couple pinches of salt and pepper along with the onion. After the onion has become translucent, toss in the garlic, cumin, and coriander. Adding the green chiles, quinoa, black beans, scallions, pepitas, feta cheese, lime juice, more salt, and pepper to taste. Mix together.
4. Stir in the diced avocado after taking the skillet from the heat and letting it cool. Adjust seasonings based on taste.
5. Fill the acorn squash halves with the filling and serve.

# 71. Butternut Squash Soup

Time: 1 hour

Serving: 8 | Calories: 600 | Fat: 24g | Carbohydrates: 70g | Protein: 23g

## Ingredients:
- ❖ 30ml Olive oil, extra virgin,
- ❖ 3g salt
- ❖ 1 large yellow onion, diced
- ❖ 3 garlic cloves, chopped,
- ❖ 1 butternut squash, peeled and cut
- ❖ 2g freshly chopped sage
- ❖ 2g freshly minced rosemary
- ❖ 3g of freshly grated ginger
- ❖ 920g of vegetable broth
- ❖ black pepper freshly ground
- ❖ 10g minced parsley
- ❖ 15g Crunchy pepitas
- ❖ Crusty bread

## Directions:
1. In a big pot, warm the oil over medium heat. Saute for 5 to 8 minutes, or until the onion is tender, adding salt as needed and plenty of freshly ground pepper.
2. Add the squash and simmer for 8 to 10 minutes, stirring periodically, until it starts to soften. Add Ginger, sage, rosemary, and garlic are added, then stir and cook for one minute or until fragrant.
3. Add three cups of the broth and increase heat. Cover and simmer. Cook for 20 to 30 minutes, or until the squash is soft.
4. Let the soup cool slightly before pouring it into a blender. If necessary, blend the soup in batches. Add up to 1 cup more broth and mix your soup if it is too thick. Serve with pepitas, parsley, and crusty bread after adding seasoning to taste.

# 72. Roasted Squash Kale Salad

Time: 1 hour 15 mins

Serving: 6 | Calories: 520 | Fat: 19.8g | Carbohydrates: 45.9g | Protein: 19.9g

## Ingredients:

- 1 squash, seeded and cut into 1.5 inches long segments.
- 1 small red onion, chopped
- 1 can of rinsed and drained chickpeas
- 2 full cloves of garlic
- 15ml Extra virgin olive oil, plus more for drizzling,
- 15ml of lemon juice, fresh

- freshly ground black pepper and sea salt
- 6 lacinato kale leaves, thinly sliced
- 200g of farro cooked
- 20g dried cranberries
- 1 gala apple, diced

## For the Pepitas maple tahini sauce:

- 15g tahini
- 5ml apple cider vinegar
- 20ml maple syrup

- 45ml of warm water; add more if necessary
- freshly ground black pepper and sea salt

## Directions:

1. Put two baking pans in the oven and preheat it to 400 degrees Fahrenheit. Put the chickpeas on one pan and the squash, red onion, and garlic cloves on the other. Olive oil and few pinches of salt and pepper should be added before tossing. Roast for 25 to 30 minutes, or until golden brown.
2. To make tahini sauce, Stir together the tahini, apple cider vinegar, maple syrup, water, and a few grinds of salt and pepper in a small bowl. Add more water while stirring to thin out the sauce if it is too thick. Allow it to settle for a few minutes to thicken if it's too thin.
3. Combine the 1/2 tbsp of olive oil, the lemon juice, and a couple pinches of salt and pepper in a sizable mixing basin. Peel the garlic cloves that have been roasted, then mash them into the combination of olive oil.
5. When the kale is barely wilted and soft, add it and give it a gentle massage. Farro and a heavy spray of tahini sauce are stirred in. Add the apple, cranberries, pepitas, red onions, chickpeas, and roasted delicata squash. Dressing may be increased if desired. Season to taste.

# 73. Rhubarb Crumble in a flash

Time: 1 hour

Serving: 4 | Calories: 180 | Fat: 13.8 g | Carbohydrates: 8.7 g | Protein: 6.7g

## Ingredients:
### *Topping:*
- ❖ Flax seed, 45g
- ❖ chopped walnuts, 15g

- ❖ Maple syrup, 60g
- ❖ 5ml vanilla extract

### *Filling:*
- ❖ Frozen apple juice concentrate, 210g
- ❖ Sliced rhubarb, 360g

- ❖ Cornstarch, 40g
- ❖ Maple syrup, 60g

## Directions:
1. Set the oven's temperature to 150 °C. Use an electric coffee grinder or a hand grinder to grind the flaxseed for the topping. Put it in a bowl and Mix well before adding the nuts, maple syrup, and vanilla extract.
2. Spread the mixture out on a cookie sheet, then toast it in the oven for 5 minutes.
3. Put the apple juice concentrate in a heavy-bottomed saucepan to make the filling. Put the rhubarb in. Rhubarb should be cooked until tender over medium heat (10 to 15 minutes). Stir in the cornstarch into the maple syrup to dissolve it. Until the mixture thickens. When the mixture is set, continuously whisk it into the rhubarb. Cut the heat.
4. Serve

# 74. Matcha Strawberry-Banana Smoothie

Time: 10 mins

Serving: 4 | Calories: 400 | Fat: 5g | Carbohydrates: 57g | Protein: 27g

**Ingredients:**
- 60g of infant spinach
- 1 matcha powder packet
- 2 bananas, medium-sized
- 1 scoop of plant protein
- 230g of almond milk without sugar

**Directions:**
1. Prior to adding the strawberries and bananas, combine the almond milk, matcha, and spinach and blend.
2. Add the remaining ingredients and blend.
3. Serve chilled

# 75. Green tea with Avocado Smoothie

Time: 10 mins

Serving: 4 | Calories: 356 | Fat: 18g | Carbohydrates: 47g | Protein: 9g

**Ingredients:**

- 1/2 an avocado
- 1 apple, coarsely cut
- 1 small zucchini, chopped
- 1/2 broccoli florets, chopped
- Grated ginger, half
- 10g of parsley, packed loosely
- 1/2 lime, juiced
- 10g cup of chopped kale
- 110g Green tea, steeped and cooled
- 230g Unsweetened almond milk
- 3g chia seeds
- Ice cubes

**Directions:**

1. Add all the ingredients into the blender jar except the chia seeds and blend till smooth.
2. Pour into a cup and sprinkle your chia seeds on the top.
3. Enjoy!

# 76. Green tea smoothie with turmeric

Time: 10 mins

Serving: 4 | Calories: 395 | Fat: 10.9g | Carbohydrates: 30g | Protein: 7.7g

**Ingredients:**

- ❖ 1g Matcha green tea powder
- ❖ 1g turmeric
- ❖ 1/2 medium banana
- ❖ 1/2 medium sized avocado
- ❖ 15g Fresh spinach,
- ❖ 115ml unsweetened almond milk
- ❖ 20g agave
- ❖ 4 cubes of ice (optional)

**Directions**:

1. Add all the ingredients to the blender, except the milk and blend.
2. Add half cup of unsweetened almond milk and blend.
3. Pour into a cup and enjoy!

# 77. Tofu Stir fry

Time: 1 hour

Serving: 4 | Calories: 297 | Fat: 17 g | Carbohydrates: 12 g | Protein: 22g

**Ingredients**:

- 340g extra-firm tofu;
- 18g low-sodium soy sauce
- 3 big garlic cloves, minced
- 1 small bunch of green onions, chopped
- 6g freshly minced ginger

- 1g fresh chili paste
- 280g Baby spinach
- 6g Toasted sesame seeds
- 10ml Sesame oil,

**Directions:**

1. Drain the tofu. Each block should be wrapped in two layers of paper towels, patted dry, and lightly squeezed to remove any remaining moisture. Tofu should be cut into 3/4-inch chunks.
2. Melt the canola oil in a sizable nonstick skillet over medium-high heat. Add the tofu and 1 tablespoon soy sauce once the oil is hot but not smoking. Be careful, as the oil will slightly splatter. For 8 to 10 minutes, or until the tofu is beautifully browned on all sides and the moisture has cooked off, sauté while stirring approximately every minute. You don't have to stir all the time. The tofu will only brown if it is left to sit for a long on one side.
3. Add the remaining 2 tablespoons of soy sauce, the ginger, garlic, about two-thirds of the green onion, and the chili paste. For about a minute, stir and cook until aromatic.
4. In order to fit more spinach in the pan, add several generous handfuls at a time, stirring as you go. Continue adding and wilting the spinach by handfuls once the initial addition has finished wilting. It will initially seem absurdly large, but it will shrink down significantly.
5. Add the sesame seeds and stir. Add the sesame oil and stir. Turn off the heat.
6. Top with the green onions. Serve hot with brown rice, noodles, or other side dish, along with a few dashes of more soy sauce and, if desired, chili paste.

# 78. Spicy Sesame Zoodles with Crispy Tofu

Time: 45 mins

Serving: 4 | Calories: 280 | Fat: 26.2 g | Carbohydrates: 11.9 g | Protein: 12.2g

## Ingredients:
### For Sriracha Sesame Sauce:

- 140g cup of peanut butter
- 30 ml of sesame oil
- 70g cup light soy sauce with low sodium
- 60g cup rice vinegar

- 6g Chili paste,
- 12g of sugar
- 1 minced garlic clove
- 1 fresh ginger knob, grated after being peeled

### For the Zoodles, and Tofu

- 340g Extra-firm tofu,
- 6 medium sized zucchinis

- onions and sesame seeds to garnish

## Directions:

1. Put all the sauce ingredients in a food processor and pulse it. Put your blended sauce in the refrigerator if you plan to serve this cold.
2. Squeeze off any extra moisture of your Tofu. Make the pieces bite-sized.
3. In a nonstick pan, heat a tiny amount of oil. Stir-fry the tofu after adding it until it turns golden. About 1/2 cup of sauce should be added, and the sauce should be simmered until it begins to evaporate or absorb into the tofu and turns brown in the pan. After some time, the tofu should be nicely golden brown with some tiny delicious browned bits from the sauce. Continue gently flipping and scraping browned bits off the bottom.
4. Prepare your zoodle by spiraling your zucchini and add roughly 1/4 cup of sauce. Add tofu, sesame seeds, and scallions as garnish. Serve right away.

# 79. Roasted Veggie Buddha Bowl with Quinoa and Avocado
### Time: 2 hours

Serving: 4 | Calories: 755 | Fat: 48 g | Carbohydrates: 64 g | Protein: 28g

**Ingredients:**
### For the Quinoa and the Buddha Bowl:
- ❖ 120g uncooked quinoa
- ❖ 20 g chopped broccoli florets
- ❖ 1/2 medium-sized head of cauliflower, chopped
- ❖ 20g broccoli
- ❖ 1 medium red onion, sliced rings
- ❖ 30ml Olive oil extra virgin
- ❖ 3g of kosher salt

- ❖ 0.5g of Black pepper,
- ❖ 340g extremely firm tofu
- ❖ 2 ripe avocados
- ❖ Sliced cucumbers, toasted pistachios, extra fresh mint, and parsley (optional additions for serving).

### For the tahini dressing:
- ❖ 15g well-stirred tahini
- ❖ 60g freshly squeezed lemon juice,
- ❖ 45g of fresh mint leaves,

- ❖ 15g of fresh parsley leaves,
- ❖ 2g of kosher salt
- ❖ 1g of Black pepper

**Directions:**
1. Boil one and half cups of water. Add the quinoa and 1/2 teaspoon of kosher salt. Once again, bring to a boil, cover, then lower heat and simmer for 12 minutes, or until the majority of the liquid has been absorbed. With a fork, remove from the heat, then cover and allow stand for 15 minutes.
2. Oven racks should be placed in the upper and lower thirds of the oven while it is preheated to 205 degrees Celsius. Place the tofu between two kitchen towels and set it on a platter while the quinoa cooks and the oven heats. Squeeze as much water as you can out of the Tofu. Transfer it into a single layer on a baking Pan that has been lined with parchment paper after being diced into 3/4-inch cubes.
3. Olive oil should be drizzled over the broccoli, cauliflower, and onion that are placed on a second baking pan. Season it with black pepper and 1/2 teaspoon salt. Put your oven's two baking pans inside and bake the vegetables for about 25 minutes, until they are soft and caramelized, and the tofu for about 20 minutes, until it is dry and firm. At the halfway point, turn the vegetables over, and switch the pan's top and bottom rack positions. Place aside.
4. Make the dressing while the tofu and vegetables are cooking. Put the tahini, lemon juice, mint, parsley, salt, and pepper, along with 1/2 cup water, in the bowl of a food processor or blender. Blend to a smooth consistency.
5. Put all the ingredients for the tahini dressing into a blender or food processor and pulse it. Then set aside.
6. When the tofu has finished cooking, let it cool slightly before putting it in a bowl with 1/4 cup of the tahini dressing and gently tossing to coat.

7. In a bowl, add the quinoa, roasted vegetables, tofu that has been dressed, and avocado. You can also add cucumber, almonds, and more fresh mint or parsley, if you like. Any leftover dressing should be served on the side for dipping or spooning, if desired.

# 80. Thai Coconut Curry Tofu

Time: 30 mins

Serving: 4 | Calories: 171 | Fat: 12.1g | Carbohydrates: 14.5 g | Protein: 10g

## Ingredients:

- ❖ 1 package extra-firm tofu, cubed after draining
- ❖ 15ml of avocado oil
- ❖ 12g Thai red curry paste
- ❖ 340g coconut milk can
- ❖ 10g soy sauce (gluten-free if needed)
- ❖ 15g of coconut sugar (substitute with maple syrup or honey)
- ❖ 1/2 lime, juiced
- ❖ 2g paprika (optional)
- ❖ cilantro and rice for serving.

## Directions:

1. A sizable nonstick pan with medium-high heat is used to heat the oil.
2. Tofu should be added to the pan and cooked for 3 to 4 minutes until golden brown on each side.
3. In a different saucepan, heat the oil over medium-high heat. Add the curry paste and cook, stirring constantly, for 30 seconds. Stirring continuously as the mixture boils for 3 to 4 minutes will cause the sauce to gradually thicken.
4. Reduce the heat to low, then stir in the paprika, soy sauce, coconut sugar, lime juice, and lime zest. Taste and adjust the seasoning.
5. Combine the curry sauce in the pan with the cooked tofu. Serve with fresh cilantro with rice.

# 81. Fluffy Silken Tofu Pancakes

Time: 45 mins

Serving: 4 | Calories: 210 | Fat: 14.6g | Carbohydrates: 19.9g | Protein: 16g

## Ingredients

- ❖ 360g of spelt flour
- ❖ 6g Baking powder
- ❖ 2g Cinnamon
- ❖ 2g of salt
- ❖ 450g Silken tofu
- ❖ 230g of your favorite non-dairy milk
- ❖ 60g Vegetable oil
- ❖ 30ml of maple syrup
- ❖ 10ml of Vanilla extract
- ❖ 60g cacao nibs

## Directions:

1. Combine the dry ingredients; flour, baking powder, salt, and cinnamon in a small basin.
2. Blend the tofu until smooth in a blender or food processor. Add the milk, vanilla, maple, and oil and blend again until smooth.
3. Gradually mix in the dry ingredients into the blended portion. It will be a rather thick batter.
4. Grease a griddle or skillet and add about 1/4 cup of batter. Cook on medium. Add some cacao nibs on top.
5. Cook the batter for about five minutes, or until the edges start to brown. To see if it is firm enough to flip, test it with a spatula. If it is, gently turn over, then heat until the other side is just beginning to brown. Add additional cacao nibs and maple syrup over top.

# 82. Scrambled Tofu

Time: 20 mins

Serving: 4 | Calories: 121 | Fat: 6 g | Carbohydrates: 7 g | Protein: 10g

## Ingredients:

- 1 garlic clove, minced.
- 1/4 red bell pepper,
- 1/2 red onion,
- 1 pack of extra firm tofu
- 10ml extra virgin olive oil
- 4g of nutritional yeast flakes
- 6g McKay's vegan chicken style seasoning
- 1g teaspoon turmeric
- salt to taste.

## Directions:

1. In a frying pan or skillet, combine your chopped onion, bell pepper, and garlic. Heat the pan or skillet over medium-high heat. When your onions become fragrant, turn off the heat.
2. Crumble the tofu and combine with the seasonings in a bowl. Place a skillet or frying pan on your stovetop over medium-high heat and add 1 teaspoon of olive oil to the bottom. Place your tofu on top of the olive oil. Stir your tofu about once per minute or so until the edges start to become somewhat firm.
3. Add the tofu into the onion-pepper mixture gently. Enjoy! Serve hot! You can eat this with salsa and some whole wheat tortillas.

# 83. Avocado Chickpea Salad Collard Wraps

Time: 15 mins

Serving: 4 | Calories: 240 | Fat: 10.3g | Carbohydrates: 27g | Protein: 11.3g

## Ingredients:

- 1 mature avocado
- 180g rinsed and drained chickpeas
- 1 medium stalk celery, diced
- 1/2 big bell pepper
- 1 lemon, juiced
- 1 medium carrot
- 10g of cilantro
- six collard greens
- salt and black pepper to taste

## Directions:

1. Mash the avocado in a large bowl. In a different bowl, add your Chickpeas and thoroughly mashed using a fork or potato masher.
2. Pour in the carrot, bell pepper, and celery. Add salt, pepper, cilantro, mashed avocado, lemon juice, and toss everything together.
3. On a chopping board, place a collard leaf flat. 1/3 cup of chickpea salad should be placed in the middle of the leaf. Then fold the leaf up like a burrito by tucking the edges under.
4. Continue until all of the chickpea salad has been consumed. Store in the refrigerator in an airtight container. Can last up to five days.

# 84. Caesar Salad with Cashew Dressing & Tofu "Croutons"
### Time: 1 hour

Serving: 4 | Calories: 251 | Fat: 15.9 g | Carbohydrates: 13.8 g | Protein: 15.9g

## Ingredients:
- 30g raw cashews
- 45ml of water
- 30ml Lemon juice
- 20g Dijon mustard

- 20g Flaxseed,
- 15g anchovy paste
- 15g Worcestershire sauce,
- 1g of garlic powder

### For the Tofu "Croutons"
- 0.5g of salt
- 1 pack extra-firm tofu, drained, and cut into 3/4-inch cubes.
- 30g of Lemon juice
- 1/4 cup Worcestershire sauce,
- 2g of powdered garlic
- 2g of powdered onion

- 45ml of olive oil
- 240g romaine lettuce, chopped
- 1 English cucumbers, thinly sliced
- 1 fresh parsley, finely chopped
- 30g of scallions, thinly sliced
- 28g Shaved Parmesan cheese.

## Directions:
1. To make dressing; Put the cashews in a small bowl and cover with boiling water. Spend at least 30 minutes soaking it.
2. Drain the cashews and add them to a blender with 3 tablespoons of water, 2 tablespoons of lemon juice, flaxseed, mustard, and anchovy paste. Blend until smooth. Place aside.
3. In the meantime, Place the tofu between sheets of paper towels on a baking pan. Place a heavy can on top, cover with another pan, and allow it drain for 15 minutes.
4. In a big bowl, combine lemon juice, Worcestershire sauce, garlic powder, and onion powder. Toss the tofu in the mixture to coat. Allow to sit for 15 minutes. Transfer the tofu to a plate.
5. Heat 1 1/2 tablespoons of oil in a sizable cast-iron skillet over medium heat. Gradually add your Tofu in two batches and cook each batch for 6 to 8 minutes, or until brown and crisp on all sides.
6. Mix the romaine, cucumber, parsley, and scallions in a large bowl to make the salad. Add the salad as dressing, on top of the crispy Tofu. Add Parmesan and the tofu "croutons" on top.

# 85. Mushroom & Tofu Stir-Fry

Time: 15 mins

Serving: 4 | Calories: 171 | Fat: 13.1g | Carbohydrates: 8.6 g | Protein: 7.7g

## Ingredients:

- 60g of canola oil
- 450g of sliced mixed mushrooms
- 1 chopped medium red bell pepper
- 1 bunch Scallions, trimmed, and diced
- 6g freshly grated ginger
- 1 big clove of grated garlic
- 230g carton of diced baked tofu
- 45g of oyster sauce

## Directions:

1. In a sizable cast-iron skillet or wok with a flat bottom, heat 2 tablespoons of oil over high heat.
2. Add the bell pepper and mushrooms; simmer for 4 minutes, stirring occasionally, until tender. Add the scallions, ginger, and garlic, and sauté for an additional 30 seconds. Place the veggies in a bowl.
3. Tofu and the remaining 2 tablespoons of oil are added to the pan. Cook for 3 to 4 minutes, turning once, until golden. Oyster sauce and the vegetables are poured in. Cook for a minute while stirring continuously.
4. Serve.

# 86. Copycat Chipotle Sofritas

Time: 35 mins

Serving: 4 | Calories: 180 | Fat: 12.7g | Carbohydrates: 10.6g | Protein: 9g

## Ingredients:

- ❖ 1 box of extra-firm tofu, drained
- ❖ 30g Tomato paste
- ❖ 20g Adobo sauce
- ❖ 3 medium garlic cloves grated
- ❖ 9g of cumin powder
- ❖ 1g dried Mexican oregano,
- ❖ 1g. of chili powder
- ❖ 45ml Extra virgin olive oil
- ❖ 1 of a medium sized yellow onion, finely chopped
- ❖ 120ml of water
- ❖ 30ml lime juice
- ❖ 1g of salt

## Directions:

1. Wrap the tofu with paper towels and squeeze gently over the sink to drain as much extra water as you can. Tofu should be put into 2-inch pieces.
2. In a small bowl, combine tomato paste, adobo sauce, garlic, cumin, oregano, and chili powder; put aside.
3. In a sizable nonstick skillet, heat the oil over medium-high heat. Add the tofu and cook for 12 minutes, sometimes flipping, until well-browned on two to three sides.
4. Add the onion and sauté it for about 3 minutes, stirring often. Stir in the tomato paste mixture after adding it. Over high heat, add water and bring to a simmer on low heat.
5. Simmer the tofu for about 4 minutes, while tossing frequently and breaking the tofu into bite-sized pieces with a spoon, until it has absorbed most of the sauce. Salt and lime juice are added after the heat is turned off.
6. Serve

# 87. Miso Soup with Veggies

Time: 30 mins

Serving: 4 | Calories: 208 | Fat: 4.4 g | Carbohydrates: 26.1 g | Protein: 17.8g

## Ingredients:

- ❖ 280g of water
- ❖ 370g of brown rice
- ❖ 60g of frozen stir-fry vegetables
- ❖ 340g extra-firm, cubed silken tofu
- ❖ 30g miso
- ❖ 2 finely scallions
- ❖ 1 teaspoon rice vinegar
- ❖ 1/2 teaspoons of sugar, or as desired

## Directions:

1. In a big saucepan over high heat, bring 2 cups of water and the rice to a boil. Cook the rice 15 minutes with the lid on, on a gentle simmer, and the heat reduced.
2. Stir in the stir-fried vegetables and bring to a boil over high heat. Cook for 2 to 3 minutes, stirring periodically, until the vegetables are well cooked.
3. Add Tofu and cook for two minutes, then cut the heat.
4. In a small dish, mix the miso with the final 3 tablespoons of water; swirl to combine. Stir together the soup, miso mixture, scallions, vinegar, and sugar.

## 88. Cauliflower Rice Risotto with Mushrooms
Time: 20 mins

Serving: 4 | Calories: 162 | Fat: 4.4 g | Carbohydrates: 13.4 g | Protein: 7.8g

### Ingredients:
- ❖ 1 head of cauliflower
- ❖ 110g of chopped mushrooms,
- ❖ 250g coconut cream,
- ❖ 6g nutritional yeast,
- ❖ I bunch fresh parsley for garnish
- ❖ 30ml butter-flavored coconut oil.

### Directions:
1. Melt Coconut oil in a big skillet over medium-high heat. Add your garlic. When the garlic is aromatic and beginning to turn golden, add the mushrooms and cauliflower and cook for about 4 minutes, or until they are soft and gently browned.
2. Cut the heat and mix your coconut cream and nutritional yeast.
3. Add a parsley garnish and serve.

# 89. Vegan Parmesan Cauliflower Steaks over Hemp Pesto Zoodles

Time: 45 mins

Serving: 4 | Calories: 208 | Fat: 18 g | Carbohydrates: 16.1 g | Protein: 17.8g

## Ingredients:

- ❖ 50ml olive oil of Spray frying oil
- ❖ 60g uncooked cashews
- ❖ 12g Nutritional yeast
- ❖ 3g of salt
- ❖ 1g of garlic powder
- ❖ 1g of black pepper
- ❖ 15g of hemp seeds
- ❖ 3 medium zucchinis
- ❖ 1 medium head of cauliflower

- ❖ 140ml almond milk without sugar
- ❖ 1/2 Juiced lemon
- ❖ 30g cup pine nuts or walnuts
- ❖ 10g of packed fresh basil leaves
- ❖ 0.5g of salt
- ❖ 3g minced garlic
- ❖ 1g of pepper

## Directions:

1. Set the oven to 200 degrees Celsius. Grease a baking sheet very lightly with olive oil or non-stick cooking spray.
2. Cashews, nutritional yeast, salt, pepper, and garlic powder should all be put in a food processor or blender. Blend until it resembles fine sand. Add 2 tablespoons of hemp seeds and stir.
3. Cauliflower's leaves should be taken off. Cut the cauliflower into 3/4-inch vertically. 3–4 slices should be enough. Place the cauliflower on the baking sheet and add a little olive oil to each side. Each cauliflower steak will have the parmesan mixture sprinkling it on both sides.
4. Bake the cauliflower for 40 to 45 minutes, or until the edges are somewhat crispy and browned.
5. Prepare the zucchini into noodles or thin strips by spiralizing them while the cauliflower is cooking. Put in a large bowl.
6. Add 1/4 cup hemp seeds, olive oil, almond milk, lemon juice, walnuts, basil, salt, garlic, and pepper to the food processor and process until smooth. Add the sauce to the zoodle and mix thoroughly.
7. On four plates, evenly distribute the zoodles. Put a cauliflower steak on top of each.

# 90. Brown Rice Pilaf

Time: 1 hour 45 mins

Serving: 4 | Calories: 400 | Fat: 24 g | Carbohydrates: 60 g | Protein: 19g

## Ingredients:

- 180g drained and soaked brown rice
- 90g chopped mixed vegetables
- 1 large, thinly sliced onion
- 3 green chilies, sliced
- 450ml of water
- Salt as desired
- 30g Clarified butter
- 60g cooking oil
- 3 cloves
- 6g ground cardamom
- 1 cinnamon stick
- 3g of grated ginger
- 1 bay leaf
- 5 minced garlic cloves

## Directions:

1. Make a smooth paste by pulverizing ginger, garlic, and cinnamon with a little water. Set it apart.
2. On medium to high heat, warm oil and clarified butter in a large pan. Stir in the bay leaf, the cloves, and the ground cardamom and cook for a few minutes.
3. Add the ground paste, then stir and cook until the raw flavor disappears.
4. Green chiles and onions should be added and sautéed until the onions are golden brown. Add the chopped vegetables in.
5. Add in your rice and give it a short stir after adding it. To the mixture, add salt and water, and then bring to a boil.
6. Reduce to medium heat and cover the pan. Cook the rice until it's soft, the vegetables crisp-tender, and the water has been entirely absorbed.
7. Serve warm alongside onion raita.

# 91. Brown Rice Crock-Pot Jambalaya
Time: 10 hours

Serving: 4 | Calories: 350 | Fat: 21 g | Carbohydrates: 50 g | Protein: 22g

## Ingredients:
- ❖ 1 sliced Andouille sausage
- ❖ 450g frozen, deveined shrimp that has been thawed
- ❖ 450g boneless, skinless chicken breast
- ❖ 1 red bell pepper
- ❖ 1 onion; 2 celery ribs

- ❖ 1 jalapeño
- ❖ 1 minced garlic clove.
- ❖ 6g Cajun seasoning
- ❖ 830ml canned diced tomatoes
- ❖ Salt and pepper to taste
- ❖ 460g chicken stock
- ❖ 390g dried white rice

## Directions:
1. In the slow cooker, add the sausage, chicken breast, seasoning, crushed tomatoes, celery, bell pepper, onion, and jalapenos. Stir in the salt and pepper. Don't add the shrimp yet.
2. Cook the chicken stock for 6 to 8 hours on low heat.
3. During the last 30 minutes of cooking, add shrimp to the slow cooker. You may remove the shells later; don't bother doing it now.
4. Parboil your rice and drain, then add the shrimp. Rice should be served alongside the jambalaya sauce, with the shrimp shells removed before eating.

# 92. Mapo Tofu

Time: 25 mins

Serving: 5 | Calories: 196 | Fat: 16.8 g | Carbohydrates: 5.7 g  | Protein: 6.7g

## Ingredients:

- ❖ 90ml canola oil.
- ❖ 20g chili bean paste
- ❖ 12g chopped, fermented black beans
- ❖ 6g of crushed red pepper
- ❖ 6g cornstarch
- ❖ 10ml of water
- ❖ 60g Lean ground beef
- ❖ 230g of low-sodium chicken broth or water
- ❖ 8g soy sauce with reduced sodium
- ❖ 1 bunch Scallions chopped into pieces,
- ❖ 430g silken tofu, drained and cut into 3/4-inch pieces.
- ❖ 1g freshly ground Sichuan peppercorns

## Directions:

1. In a small bowl, mix 5 tablespoons of oil, chili bean paste, fermented black beans, and red pepper flakes.
2. In another tiny bowl, combine cornstarch and water and whisk. Place both by the stove.
3. In a sizable flat-bottomed wok or cast-iron skillet, heat the remaining 1 tablespoon oil over medium-high heat until it shimmers. Add the beef and heat for 3 minutes or until it is thoroughly cooked and browned, breaking up the meat with a wooden spoon. Place in a compact bowl.
4. Add the saved chili bean paste mixture to the pan and heat for approximately a minute, stirring occasionally, until aromatic. Add scallions, soy sauce, and water (or broth).
5. Return the meat to the pan, then add the tofu. Cook for about 2 minutes, while gently tossing the tofu in the sauce. Stirring frequently, gradually add the cornstarch slurry, and boil for approximately a minute, or until the sauce thickens.
6. Transfer into a serving bowl, then top with ground Sichuan peppercorns.

# 93. Green Bean and Egg Salad with Garlic Parmesan Vinaigrette

Time: 25 mins

Serving: 4 | Calories: 230 | Fat: 16.3 g | Carbohydrates: 17.4 g | Protein: 2.5g

## Ingredients:

- ❖ 360g Spring Mix
- ❖ 14g fresh green beans
- ❖ 6 hard-boiled eggs
- ❖ 6 slices of cooked bacon
- ❖ 1 small red onion
- ❖ 120g of crispy croutons
- ❖ 30g grated Parmesan cheese
- ❖ 45ml of extra virgin olive oil

- ❖ 30ml white vinegar
- ❖ 15ml fresh lemon juice
- ❖ 6g Dijon mustard
- ❖ 1 minced garlic clove
- ❖ Salt and freshly ground pepper to taste
- ❖ 110g of water

## Directions:

1. In a sizable salad dish, add lettuce. Green beans should be cooked for 3 minutes after being added to boiling water in a big saucepan.
2. Drain green beans and then thoroughly rinse with ice-cold water.
3. Ads green beans to the lettuce, add croutons, sliced eggs, crumbled bacon, sliced onions.
4. Get the salad dressing ready. In a different bowl, thoroughly mix Parmesan cheese, olive oil, vinegar, lemon juice, mustard, garlic, salt, and pepper. Add one to two teaspoons of water and whisk until combined.
5. Add the dressing to the vegetables and mix well. Serve

# 94. Crispy Baked Green Bean Fries with Creamy Sriracha Sauce

Time: 30 mins

Serving: 4 | Calories: 93 | Fat: 2g | Carbohydrates: 15 g | Protein: 4g

## Ingredients:

- ❖ 28g green beans
- ❖ 2 big eggs
- ❖ 59g Panko breadcrumbs
- ❖ 2g powdered garlic
- ❖ 1g Smoked paprika
- ❖ 140g plain Greek yogurt
- ❖ 7g Sriracha,

- ❖ 1 teaspoon of shallots, minced
- ❖ 1g of smoked paprika
- ❖ 1 minced garlic clove
- ❖ 2ml of honey
- ❖ pepper and salt to taste

## Directions:

1. Set the oven's temperature to 220 degrees Celsius. Coat your baking sheet.
2. Add panko, garlic powder, and 1/4 teaspoon smoked paprika to a small bowl. Stir. Place aside.
3. Break eggs into a different small bowl and whisk to mix. Place aside.
4. Dip green beans in egg mixture and then panko mixture. To make sure the panko mixture stays, press it firmly onto the green beans. Place green beans in a single layer on a baking pan after coating.
5. Bake the crispy food for 10 to 12 minutes. In the meantime, to make our Sriracha sauce, combine the Greek yogurt, siracha, shallots, garlic, honey, smoked paprika, and salt and pepper to taste in a small bowl. Mix the combination.
6. Serve sriracha sauce with green bean fries.

# 95. Scallops with Chimichurri

Time: 45 mins

Serving: 4 | Calories: 200 | Fat: 11g | Carbohydrates: 21g | Protein: 17.8g

## Ingredients:

- 110ml of salted water
- 30ml red wine vinegar
- 1 cup chopped fresh parsley
- 2 minced garlic cloves
- A pinch of red pepper flakes
- 45ml of olive oil
- 28g of big sea scallops
- Group black pepper to taste

## Directions:

1. In a bowl, combine the water and half a teaspoon of salt. Heat for 30 seconds. After fully dissolving the salt with a stirring motion, combine the vinegar, parsley, garlic, and pepper flakes.
2. Add 2 tablespoons of the olive oil gradually while whisking to combine. The chimichurri can be used right away, but it's best to let the flavors sit for at least 20 minutes. It will keep covered in the refrigerator for 3 days.
3. In a big skillet over medium-high heat, heat the last tablespoon of oil. Use paper towels to completely dry the scallops before seasoning both sides with salt and pepper.
4. Scallops should be added to the hot oil and cooked for 2 to 3 minutes on the first side, without moving them, until a deep brown crust has formed. Cook for an additional 1 to 2 minutes on the other side, or until firm but yielding to the touch.
5. Serve with chimichurri drizzled over top.

# 96. Cornmeal Catfish With Tomato Gravy

Time: 1 hour

Serving: 4 | Calories: 340 | Fat: 16 g | Carbohydrates: 27g | Protein: 20g)

## Ingredients:

- 30ml bacon fat.
- 100g of ground cornmeal
- 430g whole, skinned tomatoes that have been lightly crushed; juices removed
- Salt and black pepper to taste
- 5ml canola oil
- 1g of cayenne
- 4 (170g each) Catfish fillets

## Directions:

1. In a medium saucepan over low heat, melt the bacon grease.
2. Then, add 2 tablespoons of cornmeal and cooked for about 5 minutes while constantly stirring.
3. Simmer for a further 10 minutes after adding the drained tomatoes. Add salt and black pepper to taste.
4. Prepare the catfish while the sauce is simmering: Over medium heat, warm the oil in a sizable cast-iron skillet or nonstick pan. Spread the cayenne pepper, a couple generous pinches of salt, and black pepper over the 1/2 cup of cornmeal in a shallow dish. Mix them together.
5. The catfish is placed in the heated pan after being dusted in the cornmeal mix on both sides.
6. Cook for 6 to 8 minutes, flipping once, or until the surface is golden brown and crusty and the fish flakes easily when you press your finger gently into it.
7. Serve. Give each fish a generous scoop of tomato gravy to dip it in.

# 97. Shrimp and Quinoa salad

Time: 35 mins

Serving: 4 | Calories: 310 | Fat: 17.8 g | Carbohydrates: 31 g | Protein: 24.6g

## Ingredients:

- lemon slices in water
- 1 bay leaf
- 12 shelled shrimp
- 1 garlic clove
- 60g dried quinoa
- 5ml olive oil
- 1/8 of a medium red pepper
- 6 cherry tomatoes
- 1/3 boiled green peas
- Ground black pepper

## Directions:

1. In a sizable stockpot over medium heat, add water, lemon slices, and a bay leaf. Bring to a boil, then let simmer for five minutes.
2. Add the raw shrimp, stir, then turn off the heat. Let the shrimp sit for about 4 minutes, or until they are all fully cooked. Peel and pour the shrimp and liquid into a colander to strain.
3. In a big skillet over medium heat, garlic and bell pepper should be stir fried in oil until they are soft. Add the shrimp after the quinoa, grape tomatoes, green peas, salt, and black pepper have been added and cook for another 5 minutes.
4. Serve hot!

# 98. Hummus recipe with fish

Time: 30 mins

Serving: 5 | Calories: 430 | Fat: 26 g | Carbohydrates: 19.8 g | Protein: 17g

## Ingredients:

- 110g Salmon filet
- 5ml of olive oil
- salt and pepper to taste
- 2 slices of lemon
- 110g boiled chickpeas
- 60g of peas, cooked,

- 7 mint leaf
- 28g Greek yogurt
- 1 spinach
- 2 radishes
- 1 tablespoon lemon juice

## Directions:

1. Set the oven to 180 degrees Celsius.
2. Place the fillet in an oven tray, top with lemon slices, sprinkle salt and pepper over the top, and drizzle with oil. After the fillet is nearly done, bake for another 13–15 minutes.
3. Mix the mint, chickpeas, peas, yogurt, and oil in a food processor. Set aside after seasoning to taste.
4. On a plate, combine the spinach and radishes. Drizzle with lemon juice, salt and pepper.
5. Serve the fillet with the pea and mint hummus.

# 99. Mashed cod and beans

Time: 45 mins

Serving: 4 | Calories: 390 | Fat: 21g | Carbohydrates: 25.4 g | Protein: 19.6g

## Ingredients:

- ❖ 5 medium tomatoes, sliced
- ❖ 5ml of olive oil
- ❖ 150g of cod fish
- ❖ salt and pepper to taste
- ❖ 10g lemon zest

- ❖ 140g cooked white beans
- ❖ 1 Garlic clove
- ❖ 15ml lemon juice
- ❖ 6 leaves of basil

## Directions:

1. Preheat the oven to 200 degrees Celsius.
2. Place the tomatoes on a baking sheet, season with salt and pepper, and drizzle with a little oil. Place the cod fish on the tray, sprinkle with extra pepper and the majority of the lemon zest, and then add a little more oil.
3. Roast the cod for 8 to 10 minutes, until it flakes easily.
4. While this is going on, place the beans, basil, lemon juice, garlic, and the remaining oil in a food processor. Pulse until a thick, slightly rough purée forms.
5. Serve the fish over the tomatoes and mashed potatoes on plates, then top with the remaining lemon zest and basil leaves.

# 100. Baby peas, salmon, and bow ties

Time: 45 mins

Serving: 4 | Calories: 208 | Fat: 13.7 g | Carbohydrates: 16.1 g | Protein: 19g

## Ingredients:

- 230g Bow tie pasta
- Quarter a big garlic clove
- 270g Silken tofu
- 220g Soy milk
- 12g freshly sliced dill

- 40g Fresh or frozen peas,
- 230g skinless salmon, cut into strips of 1 inch.
- 170g of Dijon mustard
- Pepper and salt

## Directions:

1. Add water to a pan and place it on your stovetop. Add your bowtie pasta and bring to a boil.
2. The sauce should be made while the pasta is cooking. Insert the s-blade into a food processor and add the garlic. Mince. Put the tofu in. until smooth, process.
3. Pour the tofu mixture into a pot. Add the salmon, peas, dill, and soy milk. Cook over medium heat without boiling them until they are done. Cut the heat. Add the mustard and mix. To taste, add salt and pepper.
4. The pasta is drained and rinsed. Pour the sauce over each serving of pasta at the table after placing it in a separate bowl with the sauce.

# 101. Risotto with Mushrooms
### Time: 1 hour 20 mins

Serving: 4 | Calories: 190 | Fat: 11.1g | Carbohydrates: 10 g | Protein: 9g

## Ingredients:

- 320g of water
- 120g brown rice with short grains
- A little spraying oil
- 1 sliced onion
- 3 garlic cloves, chopped
- 280g Sliced mushrooms
- 15g Brown miso
- 2g ground cumin
- 270g silken tofu
- 30g Flax seed

## Directions:

1. In a heavy-bottomed pot, bring your water to a boil. Put the rice in. Simmer the heat down. Cook for 50 minutes with a cover on.
2. Coat a large frying pan with a little spraying oil. Over a medium-high heat, heat the pan. Pour in the mushroom, onion, and garlic and brown them.
3. Add the cooked rice and stir after lowering the heat.
4. Use the s-blade attachment on a food processor to combine the miso, cumin, and tofu to Puree. Add it to the mixture of rice and mushrooms. Stir.
5. Flake in the flaxseed. Cook without boiling for 5 minutes with the lid off. Cut the heat and allow it to cool. Serve.

# JOURNAL

_____

_____

_____

_____

_____

_____

_____

_____

_____

_____

_____

_____

_____

_____

Printed in Great Britain
by Amazon

19114850R00079